PRAISE FOR
RAISING FIT KIDS IN A FAT WORLD

As always, Jesus is our role model. "He grew in wisdom and stature, in favor with God and man." We're supposed to raise our kids the same way, and this book will help enormously.

Pat Boone
Legendary entertainer and Co-author of *The Culture-wise Family*

Judy and Joani not only present the "how to" principles regarding physical fitness but also make sure parents understand the underlying factors that are necessary to genuinely help their children. I know of no book that is timelier than this extremely thoughtful yet practical book.

Ross Campbell, M.D.
Author of the bestselling books *How to Really Love Your Child*,
How to Really Parent Your Child and numerous others

Do you want your child to be free of the physical and emotional pain of obesity? This book offers a toolbox of skills that will equip you to teach your child how to stay healthy in body, mind and spirit. Thanks to *Raising Fit Kids in a Fat World*, my seven-year-old has learned quickly and easily how to eat what his body is calling for in the amounts his growing body needs for energy and good health!

Lisa Cauto, R.N.
Grapevine, Texas

I like the Fit Kids method because you can really eat whatever you want, as long as you stop when your tummy's full. However, I have learned that even though candy and junk food is yummy, IT DOESN'T FILL YOU UP! Parents and kids will love this book!

Jessica Jack, Age 13
Daughter of Joani Jack, M.D.

Some books are designed to be read; this one should be absorbed by the whole family. *Raising Fit Kids in a Fat World* is not about a new diet; it is about greater health for everyone. It is jam packed with so much common sense it is like "brain bran" for fresh thinking about eating. Nothing in this book is hazardous to your health. If you want a healthy approach to food in your family, I highly recommend this volume for you.

Michael S. Lawson, Ph.D.
Chairman and Senior Professor, Christian Education Department,
Dallas Theological Seminary, and Author, *Grandpa Mike Talks About God*

When I began to read *Raising Fit Kids in a Fat World*, I thought it was just another diet book that would be put on my library shelf with a bookmarker around page 20. But these qualified authors grabbed my attention with their years of experience concerning the spiritual, emotional, mental and physical needs of our children. Judy and Joani are offering some real hope that we as parents can use to raise fit kids that will enjoy a wholesome lifestyle.

Ron R. Ritchie
Free at Last! Ministry, Menlo Park, California

If I had had this book when I was raising my children, I know it would have made a difference in the way we looked at food. Every parent should read this book *before* their children arrive, but even if you are well into the parenting process, read it anyway. It will rock your world for the better!

Jan Silvious
Author, *Big Girls Don't Whine* and *Foolproofing Your Life*

Judy Halliday and Joani Jack give parents practical ways to teach children God-honoring principles of eating and drinking for life, health and enjoyment. I am convinced that following these principles will help prevent eating disorders and lead children to better health and more confident living.

Leonard Stob
Superintendent, Ontario Christian Schools, Ontario, California

RAISING
FIT KIDS
IN A FAT
WORLD

JUDY HALLIDAY, R.N.
JOANI JACK, M.D.

Regal

From Gospel Light
Ventura, California, U.S.A.

Published by Regal
From Gospel Light
www.regalbooks.com
Ventura, California, U.S.A.
Printed in the U.S.A.

Library of Congress Cataloging-in-Publication Data
Halliday, Judy.
  Raising fit kids in a fat world / Judy Halliday, Joani Jack.
    p. cm.
  Includes index.
  ISBN 978-0-8307-4534-0 (hardcover)
  1. Obesity in children—United States—Prevention. 2. Obesity in children—Religious aspects—Christianity. 3. Children—Nutrition—Religious aspects—Christianity. I. Jack, Joani. II. Title.
  RJ399.C6H32 2007
  618.92'398—dc22
                                                                        2007021804

1 2 3 4 5 6 7 8 9 10 / 10 09 08 07

Rights for publishing this book outside the U.S.A. or in non-English languages are administered by Gospel Light Worldwide, an international not-for-profit ministry. For additional information, please visit www.glww.org, email info@glww.org, or write to Gospel Light Worldwide, 1957 Eastman Avenue, Ventura, CA 93003, U.S.A.

Judy's Dedication:

To all Thin Within moms and dads
who have had the courage and faith to raise children
who are physically and spiritually fit

Joani's Dedication:

To my mom,
Edith Brown Barnes
September 4, 1932–September 20, 2006
I'm glad you are happy and healthy with Jesus
But I really, really miss you

CONTENTS

INTRODUCTION

Your toddler looks you right in the eye and emphatically screams, "No!" Your daughter walks bravely into school on the first day of kindergarten. Your son stands alone at the spelling bee podium. You turn out the light after gazing at that angelic face, sleeping peacefully. Then at 2 A.M., the night of the senior prom, the ringing phone shatters your peaceful dreams and sends your heart into your stomach! Parenting is full of ups and downs, giggles and tears, pride and shame, hopes and fears. One moment you would give up *everything you own* for that precious child. A few minutes later you feel like handing him over to the next stranger who crosses your path!

In the midst of our crazy and challenging lives looms a *huge* problem, which is steadily gaining ground. It hits us where it hurts the most by threatening the hopes and dreams we have for our children. It is called childhood obesity. Currently one out of five children is overweight, impacting nearly half the families in this country.

We wonder if the world has gone crazy! A serving from the children's menu can feed two adults. A single dinner entrée can feed the entire family. Children's clothing comes in plus sizes. Children are parked in front of the TV, missing the joy of engaging in active exercise. Everyone is concerned—doctors, coaches, dads, moms and even children themselves. Is your child one of those affected or at risk? Are you overweight and fearful that your child will follow in your footsteps? Does the very subject bring a lump to your throat or a tightening in your chest? If so, take heart . . . hope is on the way.

Raising Fit Kids in a Fat World is unlike any other approach you've encountered. It is about preventing and treating childhood obesity in a unique, time-tested way that will transform your child's life. New and exciting insights will infuse your parenting practices with clarity and confidence. Innovative ideas will help you teach your child healthy, nonfood-related ways of coping with the stress of life. You will learn how to make changes based on facts and faith—changes that will result in a child that is not only fit and trim on the outside but also joyful on the inside.

What sets our approach apart from weight-loss programs for children? We seek to help parents raise children who are healthy and whole—our approach is not just about losing weight; it's about making a lifestyle change. It's a simple, sensible way of life with a proven track record, and it can travel wherever you go—from the ball field to Disney World. And it's something that you and your child will enjoy doing!

Your child will attain his natural, God-intended size while learning to eat the right *amount* of foods and the right *kinds* of foods and becoming more consistently active. Diets cannot accomplish this—they don't work in the long run and can even be harmful for children. Rest assured you won't need to count calories or carbs, buy special foods or prepare specific menus. Instead, your child will learn to pay attention to his or her God-given cues of hunger and fullness, resulting in a decrease in the amount of food eaten—but *without* rigid or restrictive rules. At the same time, you will learn creative and effective ways to encourage wise food choices as well as increased activity.

To help your child reach her natural size, "high love" will be far more important than "low carb." Rather than prescribing strict rules, this book will encourage and equip you to interact with your child in ways that motivate personal change.

So, are you ready to teach your child the freedom of listening and responding to his body's cues for hunger and satisfaction? Discover together wonderful foods that taste sensational and pack power-filled nutrients? Enjoy new and compelling activities that will delight you and your child? Learn how to connect heart to heart with your child? Lead your child on a closer walk with God?

What do most of us *really* want for our children? We want them to do what is right, to know true love, to laugh, to believe, to take risks, to become wise, to succeed, and to know the peace of God that surpasses all understanding. We know that you love your children more than words can express. Grab hold of that love and don't abandon those dreams. You *can* raise a fit kid in a fat world, and we're here to show you how to do it.

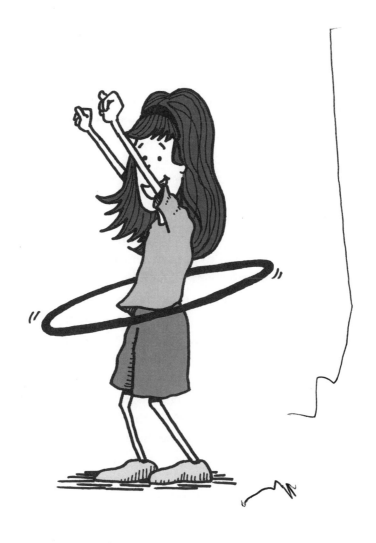

CHAPTER 1

HAVE HOPE!

An Effective Solution to a *Big* Problem

arah became obese as a toddler. She had diabetes at 7 years of age. Her first hospitalization for diabetes occurred when she was only 8. Her high blood pressure began at age 10. Her family's lack of attention to these problems led to asthma, heart problems, and scores of hospitalizations. Finally, at age 14, Sarah's body gave out. Her last hospital stay was for a diabetic coma that led to a massive heart attack."[1] Walt Larimore, M.D., sounds the wake-up call by publicizing this heartbreaking story.

This generation of children faces a future of unprecedented medical consequences related to obesity. Diseases previously seen only in adults, such as diabetes, high blood pressure, cholesterol abnormalities, and many others, are now occurring in children. For the first time, experts are seriously examining whether our current generation of children will have a decreased lifespan due to issues related to being overweight.[2] We are now testing for diabetes in children as young as two years of age.

In addition to the medical challenges that are part of childhood obesity, the emotional impact felt by children and families can be devastating as well. Perhaps you know this all too well. You may have an overweight child in your life—a son, a daughter, a grandchild, or someone in your circle of close friends. You may not know whether to weep, scream, pray, or run and hide! You may be desperately searching for answers for what seems like an insurmountable problem. If so, you aren't alone. Statistics indicate that *lots* of children are overweight, with one out of five now facing obesity.

In the midst of this harsh reality, we want to give you an infusion of hope. We want to turn your fears into resolve, replace your uncertainty with a clear plan, answer your confusion with the facts, and let the power of hope inspire and uplift you. Today you are invited to take the first step on the path of raising a healthy, lean, fit child, and we want you to take this journey, secure in the firm belief that this is something *you can do!*

First of all, *this is not a diet.* All of those "how to lose weight quick" ideas need to go directly into the garbage can. Ditch the food scale. Forego the low-carb versus low-fat debate. Stop counting your child's calories. You may have already discovered that diets can be expensive, frustrating, guilt-inducing and ineffective in the long run. Welcome to a refreshing, effective, time-tested alternative.

So, how do we move from propaganda and failure to an approach that will achieve the results you are looking for? The answer will become clearer with each page of this book.

Let's start at the beginning—literally: *Your child is well made.* When God finished creating humankind, He didn't say, "It's okay" or "It's not bad." Not at all. Instead, God looked at what He created and said, "It is very good" (Gen. 1:31). We suspect you believe there is no child in the world as wonderful as your own. But did you realize that your child is God's masterpiece—an awesome, intricate creation designed for health and wholeness? Our steadfast hope for your child is firmly based on this foundation.

God also created an incredible variety of nourishing foods for us to enjoy. Some foods are full of nutrients and vitamins, and others are not. Some foods taste good and others feel good. Few foods are all bad and few are all good.

Food is like fuel. Some are high quality and cost more; some are low quality and cost less (lately they all cost a lot!). While our bodies can usually run on whatever we put in the tank, we will run more efficiently and last longer with good fuel (proper nutrition) and regular maintenance (proper exercise).

Despite having well-designed bodies and quality foods readily available, we as a society are out of shape and in the midst of a health crisis. Why? The answer is a sad indictment of the American way of life. The popular media sends us so many mixed messages that we end up being thoroughly confused when it comes to understanding nutrition and the human body. Many of us aren't interested in exerting the effort required to be healthy, having been bombarded with the message that we should pursue whatever makes us feel and look good, preferably as fast as possible. We're encouraged to do whatever we want, whenever we want, and to stop whenever we darn well please. If consequences of such behaviors arise, hopefully there is a pill or some other quick fix readily available. Our culture doesn't advocate delayed gratification or self-control, whether we're talking about eating, work, relationships or shopping.

As the world around us pursues the feel-good lifestyle, our health is suffering. Quick fixes work for a short time and then trigger an inevitable breakdown. All the while our bodies are trying to send us messages that all is not well. "Hello, up there? That's enough! Could you stop shoveling in more food? Let me get a little rest. And take me out for some exercise . . . please!"

The problem is, we're too busy keeping up our frantic pace of life. It's time to *slow down*—to make the effort to point our children toward the path of health by tuning into their God-given signals of hunger and fullness. In the process, the entire family will benefit from discovering what God really intended when He brought your little masterpiece into this world.

What's the Big Deal?

While many may feel overwhelmed at the notion of attempting to deal with an overweight child, others (perhaps within the same home) may question why being obese is of such concern. We live in a wealthy country with an abundance of good food and we're all getting bigger. So let's just be "large and in charge." Make bigger clothes, bigger cars and larger refrigerators; build bigger bathrooms, bigger chairs and super-sized caskets! Be fat and happy. What's the big deal?

Consider the impact of the following words: "Fat." "Obese." "Huge." "A cow." "Overweight." "Plump." "Chunky." "Plus-sized." "Heavy." "Stout." "Extra large." These are words that can be used in many different ways—on a menu, in a movie title or in everyday conversation. Some could even be a medical description or a compliment. They don't evoke an emotional reaction or convey judgment. These are *just words*.

Yeah, right!

These are *not* just words to anyone who has ever experienced the pain of being overweight. How does our culture feel about those who are overweight? An unsettling answer to that question occurred during the Obesity Treatment and Prevention conference in Seattle, Washington, in 2004. During a lecture, the speaker passed out blank index cards to healthcare professionals and asked each person to complete the following sentence: "People who are overweight are _____." The responses were *absolutely stunning*. While a few were positive, many were negative—and some were downright mean: "Pigs." "Ugly." "Unhappy." "Hopeless." "Unmotivated." "Lazy." "Scary." "Impossible to help." And these answers came from healthcare workers who wanted to learn how to *help* those who are overweight! That being the case, can you imagine the answers a class of fourth-graders might give to the same type of question?

Well, imagine no longer. When a group of 10- and 11-year-old children were asked to study pictures of children with varying disabilities and rank them in order of acceptability, the obese child was rated below all the physical deformities, including a missing hand and facial disfigurement.[3] It gives a discouraging slant to the old saying, "I'd give my right arm to be thin." Your child, or perhaps his best friend, may indeed feel the same way. Our culture places a tremendously high priority on physical appearance.

If these two disparate groups—professional healthcare workers and elementary school students—are an indication of the prevailing opinions of our society, then our overweight children face a difficult struggle against deeply ingrained stereotypes. While we desperately wish that this weren't the case, we need to recognize the battles our overweight children are facing. It is a *very* big deal.

Your Child, God's Masterpiece

If your heart is feeling pierced, please know: God knows and cares deeply for all children and He is *crazy* about your child! Amazingly enough, He loves your child even more than you do. That's almost impossible for us to comprehend, but it is incredibly reassuring. So we ask: Who better to be in charge? Throughout this book, we will emphasize the following concept: God created your child. Let's turn to Him for help in understanding how your child's body was designed to work.

You made all the delicate, inner parts of my body and knit me together in my mother's womb. Thank you for making me so wonderfully complex! Your workmanship is marvelous—how well I know it. You watched me as I was being formed in utter seclusion, as I was woven together in the dark of the womb. You saw me before I was born. Every day of my life was recorded in your book. Every moment was laid out before a single day had passed (Ps. 139:13-16).

Your child has a bright future designed by our loving, all-knowing and all-powerful heavenly Father. Regardless of the obstacles in your path, God is on your child's side.

Picking up this book is an important beginning. You have taken the first step toward setting your child free from diets and other subtle entrapments, and you are embarking on a path of truth that will bring health and wholeness to your child.

The Fit Kids Method

Our approach is simple but not necessarily easy. It is faith-based and grace-oriented. It's not a diet, and it's not about rigid rules or harsh treatment. You will need no special food, no special recipes, no carb or calorie counters. Nor will we encourage a sudden change to making macaroni and cheese with whole-grain pasta and cheese substitutes (which six-year-old Jessica pronounced "gross"). The only "equipment" you will need is your child (and his or her brain, mouth and stomach) and your own willingness to guide her on the God-intended path to health.

Raising Fit Kids in a Fat World is based on a threefold approach called the "three senses"—*science* sense, *common* sense and *God's* sense. This approach will be woven throughout this book.

Science sense means sharing medical facts that are available from the leading experts in the field of obesity, studies from current medical literature, and our clinical experiences in counseling and treating patients. In Medical Moments, we discuss the latest findings pertaining to specific issues. Although it is our intent to provide the most accurate scientific information available, please remember that you should always rely on your pediatrician or family physician for specific medical advice.

Common sense utilizes time-tested principles that directly apply to your day-to-day life situations. Our Common Sense Corner is a place to "be real" and will teach you to raise a fit kid in the midst of a crazy, hectic, confusing world.

God's sense is the foundation that underlies everything. It is ultimate truth put into place by God our Creator, demonstrated to us by Jesus, explained to us through His divinely inspired Word and whispered to us through the Holy Spirit. Throughout the book, Spirit Moments will offer a godly perspective on many different situations.

The three senses are complementary, not contradictory. When woven together, they form a threefold bond of incredible strength and durability that you can rely on throughout your journey toward better health.

Raising Fit Kids in a Fat World will first focus on teaching your child to eat the *right amount* of food by learning to recognize his internal signals of hunger, satisfaction and fullness. Children who are overweight will begin to eat less food and, as a result, will gradually attain their appropriate, God-intended size. Children who are a normal weight will simply remain so and avoid the epidemic of inappropriate weight gain that is sweeping our nation. Your child will also learn to eat the *right types* of food by learning to choose and enjoy wise choices. We will dispel many myths associated with nutrition and look at what the medical community has to say regarding how different foods affect the body. And you and your family will learn to *be active* on a daily basis, allowing your child to drop any excess weight, improve cardiovascular health and be the fit kid that he surely wants to be. (These concepts and many more are part of the Fit Kids Triangle, which we will present in chapter 7).

One of the greatest challenges that children (and adults) face in our culture is eating the right amount of food. It's fairly obvious that children who are overweight need to eat less. But how? By counting points? Restricting calories? Calculating the glycemic load? We will examine different aspects of diets later on, but the focus for now is to teach your child to eat less without being on a rigid diet and to attain a healthy, fit size.

Think for a moment about your family's eating habits, particularly as they relate to your child. Do you tend to feed your child based on what the clock says, or based on her hunger needs? On the flip side, does the meal end when your child has finished everything on her plate, or when she is satisfied? We are all born with the natural ability to feel hunger, seek nourishment and stop eating when satisfied. But if your child gets in the habit of eating whether or not she is hungry and continues eating beyond the point of physical satisfaction, then her natural, God-given signals will be overruled, and your child will frequently choose to eat *too much* food. The result will be excessive weight gain.

Over the next few days, notice whether hunger and satisfaction even play a role in your children's desire to eat. As you become more conscious of your family's eating habits, you may become aware of mistakes you have made. If so, don't sweat it. All of us have "been there and done that." Recognizing a mistake is the first step toward correcting your course.

To help your child learn how much to eat, we will utilize two models: the young infant who instinctively knows when and how much to eat, and the naturally thin adult who maintains a healthy, God-ordained size by consistently eating only that which the body requires. As we explore these models, you will begin to appreciate the miracle of the human body. Our bodies are not perfect—we've lived in an imperfect world far too long for that—but the basic design is amazing. As your child learns to recognize and respond to the God-given sensations of hunger and satisfaction, he will begin eating the right amount of food.

As you learn more about hunger and satisfaction, it will become obvious that we often use food not to satiate physical hunger, but to meet emotional needs. We used to be taught, "When life hands you lemons, make lemonade!" Now, we are more likely to hear, "When life hands you lemons, you *owe it to yourself* to eat an entire lemon pie!" Learning to deal with emotional needs in a manner that does *not* involve food is one of our most important challenges. We face stress and temptations on a daily basis, and so do our children. When faced with difficulties—or even when celebrating success—your child can learn to turn to God, rather than to food, to meet his innermost longings.

We usually turn to God when we experience a serious illness, financial crisis, loss of a job, or a death. But if we have a "bad hair day," break up with a boyfriend, fail to make the basketball team, have dealings with a grumpy coworker or wake up to cranky kids, it's much more likely that we'll seek consolation in chips or cheesecake. We have all done it, but does it really make sense?

Teaching your child to turn to God for help with everything from the daily hassles to the life-altering catastrophes allows your child to experience God's many faces: friend, confidant, counselor, rescuer and savior. Of course, you can't give what you don't have. So if you don't feel as close to God as you would like to be, you might begin closing that gap by talking with Him daily about the little, everyday things that bother you rather than seeking Him only when a crisis occurs. He cares about every detail of our lives, listens to our every word and loves to be in relationship with you and your child. In fact, that's the reason He created each and every one of us. As you and your child draw near to God, everything else in life will begin to fall into place.

You may feel that getting involved in a faith-based weight-loss program is risky. If you mess up, will you have failed your child *and* failed God? A thousand times, *no!* Remember, God's love for you and your child *is not based on appearance, performance or success.* His love is real, pure, perfect, and there isn't anything any of us can do to change that. It is love based on His unending grace and mercy that cannot be fully understood—only enjoyed and appreciated. The more we know of His sovereignty, love, mercy and grace, the more we will want to follow His precepts and take proper care of our wonderfully made bodies.

The Madness

If we all employed a full-time cook and lived in a controlled environment with a personal trainer at our beck and call, it would be much easier for us to be fit. But for most of us, life just isn't that way! We all need to get fit and stay healthy, even in the madness of day-to-day living. For this reason, our approach to a healthy lifestyle is practical, adaptable and suitable for every facet of daily life.

To put our concepts into practice, we have designed tools to help convey specific ideas to your child.

- The Tummy Keys will help your child eat less food by showing him to pay attention to what his body is saying.

- The Belly Meter will give you a language with which to teach even a very young child to recognize when her stomach is empty, satisfied or too full.

- The Fun Jar and the Motion Monitor will help you adopt an active lifestyle with an adventurous spirit.

- Stop, Drop and Roll will address needed behavior changes within your family and equip you to make those changes a reality.

- The Word Wand will give you specific ways to better communicate with your child.

These tools will provide practical, simple ways to integrate the Fit Kids method into your child's daily life, as you begin to appreciate that preventing or treating childhood obesity involves not just nutrition, but also behavior modification, clear boundaries, good parenting skills and a great deal of commitment and prayer by the entire family.

Yet having your child come to terms with his weight-related issues can be a challenge. For this reason, underlying everything must be lots of unconditional love, honesty, wisdom, patience and perseverance. As we address behavior changes as they relate to your child, we will seek God's guidance in dealing with a variety of challenging food-related issues.

Ultimately, understanding hunger and fullness will become second nature. But there will always be obstacles lurking around the corner. Just when you think you have it under control, life happens—stress, vacations, money problems, holidays, divorce, death, and other challenges. An effective weight-loss and weight-maintenance method works during the good *and* the bad times. We plan to give you strategies to meet these inevitable and unexpected stresses in life that might otherwise defy your commitment to your child's health and fitness.

Wanting It All

A popular sweatshirt reads, "Dear Santa, I want it all." Does that ring true for you? Many of us want a loving family, a big house, the cool car, an awesome job, the best friends, and lots of great vacations thrown in for good measure.

Is it wrong to want the good life for you and your child? Not necessarily. God gave us a beautiful world to enjoy, and desiring good things for ourselves and for our families is normal. Accepting the gifts God has given us and using them wisely is appropriate. Wanting it all, however—that's another matter entirely. We live in a country that has more of everything than almost any other place on the face of the earth. Some would say we "have it all." But are we happier? Not even close. Why is that? In wanting it *all*, is it possible we have forgotten what it's really all about?

Does this hold true when it comes to our dreams for our kids? Why *do* you want your child to be fit? Is it out of love and a genuine desire for physical and emotional well-being, or is it so that the family meets the worldly requirements of outward success? Are you fostering your child's God-given gifts and talents, or are you expecting her to fulfill a dream of your own making? Are you pressuring your child to obtain unrealistic accomplishments in your attempt to have it all?

When children are raised with *high* worldly expectations and *low* levels of affirmation, they may perform to perfection outwardly, but inwardly they are forever striving for that which they cannot attain or sustain. This may lead to worsening obesity or to conditions such as anorexia/bulimia, a heartbreaking outcome for any child and one we all want to avoid.

Wanting It God's Way

There is a breathtaking alternative to the rat race that comes with wanting it all, and that is *wanting it God's way*. In today's culture this choice is the narrow path that is sometimes portrayed as backward and "un-cool." Yet those who choose it experience profound peace and contentment.

This way isn't easy—nothing worthwhile ever is. This choice begins with the recognition that our deepest longings aren't met by worldly success but by knowing God. As you seek God first, you will probably feel as though you are swimming upstream, fighting a strong "me-first," materialistic current. And yet, as you implement God's plan for your beloved child, he or she will be transformed into someone who chooses to resist temptation, looks beyond self, reaches out to those in need, and stands strong on godly principals of truth. The end result for both you and your child will be peace, contentment, joy and wisdom.

Let's Do It!

So what's it going to be? Do you want it God's way? Will you take the plunge and make the commitment to raise a spiritually and physically fit child? If so, this will be a significant turning point for you and your child, as you teach him to love the amazing body God created, to enjoy good food and to live life to the fullest. Finding freedom from the "wanting it all" rat race, rigid food rules, the me-first mentality, and the prison of obesity will be absolutely exhilarating. God's way will always be worth it, will never disappoint and will leave you more than satisfied. It's time to set your child free!

The Lifeline of Prayer

You are not alone. God knows all your cares, heartaches, joys and sorrows. Let Him take on the burden you've been carrying and infuse you with the peace that comes only from Him.

When you are faced with a melt-down situation, or when the kids are completely out of control and demanding a run to McDonald's, don't despair or give up. Instead, look up. What God desires from us more than anything else is not perfection but a *relationship* with Him. Talk to God constantly—about the good and the bad, your fears and dreams, your successes and your failures. He will lovingly guide you as He comforts you with His presence.

Father, You know the struggles we're wrestling with
and what makes us feel uncertain, scared, happy and sad
as we try our best to be good parents.
You custom made each child to be unique.
Give us Your peace as You quiet our fears
and help us believe that our children are Your masterpieces
and that You know what is best.
Help us to turn to You for all of our needs, big and small.
Thank You for Your unconditional love and amazing grace.
Grant us Your peace and help us to choose to live life Your way.
Amen.

Don't worry about anything; instead, pray about everything. Tell God what you need, and thank him for all he has done. If you do this, you will experience God's peace, which is far more wonderful than the human mind can understand. His peace will guard your hearts and minds as you live in Christ Jesus.

PHILIPPIANS 4:6-7

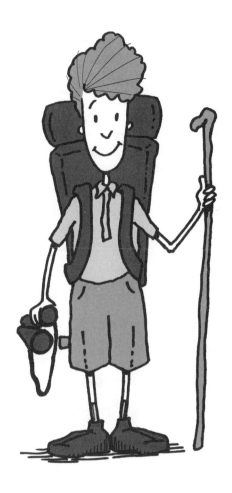

CHAPTER 2

GETTING ORIENTED

Finding Your Starting Point

Remember your last family vacation? "Daddy, I've gotta go to the bathroom!" "Are we *there* yet?" "Mom, he's *looking* at me!" Most family vacations are filled with moments of laughter, family bonding and plenty of sibling squabbles! Whether driving across the country using Mapquest to find your way, or flying with a bird's eye view of the terrain below, one thing is absolutely essential to make it a success: a clear understanding of your starting point. To get where you are going, you must understand where you *are*.

As you begin this journey, we encourage you to be totally, no-fudging, 100-percent honest! While facing the truth sometimes hurts, it is *always* a courageous, giant step forward. Human nature often screams for us to bury our heads in the sand. And yet remaining in denial is hard work! Repressing anxious thoughts about an overweight child can be tiring and stressful. A dose of honesty may remove some of that burden, bringing in its wake relief and fresh energy. An accurate assessment of where you are will provide a great start, leading to transformation and adventure.

Family History

You have likely heard it said that "the apple doesn't fall far from the tree," and studies on childhood obesity seem to bear that out. If one parent is overweight, a child is three times more likely to be overweight; two overweight parents and the child is *ten* times more likely to be overweight.[1] As children attempt to lose weight, one of the biggest factors of their success or failure is—you guessed it!—whether or not the rest of the family is on board.[2] Children are affected by the genetics of their parents, but they are equally affected by what they observe their parents doing. So, Mom and Dad, you get to join in the fun, too! Successful weight loss in kids begins with the understanding that both genetics and family environment are extremely important.

Vanessa became quite upset during a recent visit to her children's pediatrician, confiding, "My husband is very obese, and although I constantly worry about the kids and their weight, he just doesn't seem to care. He figures he's just fine, so if our children end up being overweight, it won't be that big of a deal." Vanessa struggles with the right words to convey to her husband the health hazards and negative emotional side effects of obesity. She rightfully recognizes that her children have a genetic tendency toward obesity and are also being exposed to a poor role model. Fortunately, the influence that Vanessa has in her family through her own example is a powerful and encouraging place to begin.

If Vanessa's story rings true for you, take heart: "With people this is impossible, but with God all things are possible" (Matt. 19:26, *NASB*). The one who calmed the sea and raised the dead travels with you, and He will provide all you need for the transformation you desire.

Because children are affected by both genetics and living environment, please answer the following questions for both the biological parents and other adults who may have an influence on your child. Answer the questions for each child for whom you have some concern (use separate sheets of paper for your answers, if necessary).

Health, Weight, Fitness

Mom and Dad, let's start with you. Describe your health, weight and fitness below (circle one):

Overall Health:	Awful	Fair	Pretty Good	Great
Childhood Weight:	Really big	Plump	Just Right	Too Skinny
Current Weight:	Very Overweight	Overweight	Normal	Too Thin
Fitness:	Couch Potato	Not so Fit	Fairly Fit	Fit as a Fiddle

Circle any of these that are, or have been, present within the family (parents, siblings or grandparents):

Obesity	High Blood Pressure	Heart Disease	Diabetes	High Cholesterol
Depression	Eating Disorders			

Food Habits

Please answer the following questions using a scale of 0 to 10, with "0" meaning "never" and "10" meaning "always."

How often is your child on a diet?_____

Do you "stress out" over what your child eats?_____

Do you use guilt to influence your child's food choices?_____

Do you feel overwhelmed or unprepared regarding nutrition for your child?_____

Do you worry about your child's weight?_____

Do you think your child is unattractive due to his or her weight?_____

Does your child feel unattractive?_____

Does your child think he or she is fat?_____

Do you make clothing/style choices based on your child's weight?_____

Do you make social or extracurricular activity choices based on your child's weight?_____

Can you visualize your child as trim or healthy? _____

Is food and/or your child's weight a source of conflict? _____

Do you frequently check your child's weight?_____

Do you allow your child to eat whatever and whenever he wants?_____

For the questions below, please circle the answer that best describes your situation.

When eating, are you aware of *your* body's hunger and fullness signals?
Yes, always   Sort of   No way—my body has those?

Does *your child* seem to realize when he is hungry, satisfied and full?
Definitely   Maybe   You're kidding, right?

Do *you* wait for true hunger before eating?
Always   Usually   Sometimes   Never

Does *your child* wait for true hunger before eating?
Always   Usually   Sometimes   Never

Do *you* stop eating when satisfied, before becoming too full?
Always   Usually   Sometimes   Never

Does *your child* stop eating when satisfied, before becoming too full?
Always   Usually   Sometimes   Never

Do *you* normally finish everything on your plate?
Never   Sometimes   Often   Always

Does *your child* usually finish everything on her plate?
Absolutely Not Sometimes Often Always

Does your child have to eat all of his food to get dessert?
Never Sometimes Often Always

Do you and your child have power struggles over food choices?
Never Sometimes Often At every meal

Next, imagine your stomach as a balloon and answer the following questions using a scale of 0 to 10. A "0" is when the balloon is completely empty, while a "10" is when the balloon is completely filled up to the point it is about to pop.

I normally *start* eating at a _____.
I normally *stop* eating at a _____.
My child usually *starts* eating at a _____.
My child usually *stops* eating at a _____.

Spirit Moment: Honesty

By now you've begun to get an idea of your starting place. As we evaluate our own behaviors and how they affect our kids, we might feel a bit . . . squeamish. We probably hope no one sees our answers! And yet, what God desires from us during these times is honesty.

In his letter to the Galatians, Paul says, "Make a careful exploration of who you are and the work you have been given, and then sink yourself into that. Don't be impressed with yourself. Don't compare yourself with others" (Gal. 6:4-5, *THE MESSAGE*). Not only is it very important to look at who we are and the work we have been given, but it is also important that we not worry about what others think. While the "wanting it all" approach might be preoccupied with outward success, we are going to focus on doing it God's way. That means being realistic about the work ahead and pursuing it for the right reasons.

When it comes to our kids, we parents tend to feel strongly about a lot of things. Just try to blame *our* child for starting the spit-wad fight in the school cafeteria! Denial and rationalization are often the trademarks of loving parents, but both can be major hindrances to accomplishing the task before us. Ask God to help you be honest and avoid comparisons as you boldly take a good look at reality. He will honor your honesty and your good intentions.

Food and Emotions

Perhaps one truth many of us have encountered is that our emotions affect what, how much and how fast we eat, as well as our digestion. Think about meals you had that were accompanied by strong emotions, either good or bad. Have you ever had an argument while eating? If so, how did your stomach feel? Was it an "antacid moment"? On the other hand, when you recall a special meal that was filled with love and happiness, you may be able to remember the flavor and smell of the food as well as the warm glow of the entire experience. Every emotion—the high of a job promotion, the constant chaos of lost shoes and late homework assignments, mellow feelings of peace and contentment—can affect our eating experience. In turn, how we as parents eat affects our kids. Children crave peace, order and structure, and they tend to follow nonverbal cues. As parents, we must remember: "Attitudes are caught, not taught."

Cindy's story of a meal that she and her husband shared illustrates how the entire eating experience can be altered by emotions. "While waiting for dinner to be served at our favorite restaurant, we began arguing, and it escalated throughout the meal. The only thing I remember about the food was seeing the steak through a blurry haze of tears." When she tried to recall the meal experience, the only memory that lingered was one of heartache.

Let's look at some of the emotional and environmental situations that can impact eating in your family. This exercise *isn't* designed to be a "club of condemnation" with which to beat yourself over the head. Quite the contrary! Describing your current habits will eventually help you see how far you've come. In a few months or a year, you can look back and rejoice at the positive changes that have been incorporated into your daily life. For now, however, as you respond to the questions below, you are gathering important data about what makes you and your child tick.

Answer the following questions using a scale of 0 to 10. This time, "0" means "never" and "10" means "always."

Our family eats on the run. _____
Our family eats separately rather than together. _____
Our family eats somewhere *other than* the dinner table. _____
Our family eats fast food. _____
Our family eats out at restaurants. _____
Our meals involve arguments or conflict. _____
Our family celebrates with food. _____
Our family eats for emotional reasons. _____
Family outings are planned around food. _____
My child eats due to stress or boredom. _____
My child eats because of unhappiness or sadness. _____
My child overeats in social situations (with friends,
     at parties, at sporting events, and so on). _____
My child prefers eating alone. _____
My child eats in front of the TV or computer. _____
My own bad eating habits seem to affect my child. _____

In general, how do you rate your life *in the following areas? Again,* answer using a scale of 0 to 10. "0" means terrible and "10" means wonderful.	*In general, how do you rate* your child's life *in the following areas? Again, answer using a scale of 0 to 10. "0" means terrible and "10" means wonderful.*
Overall health _____	Overall health _____
Energy level _____	Energy level _____
Self-esteem _____	Self-esteem _____
Job satisfaction (consider student or homemaker as a job) _____	Success in school and/or work _____
Outside interests _____	Talents/success in extracurricular activities _____

Marriage/romantic relationships _____	Relationships with parents _____
Relationship with your children _____	Relationships with siblings _____
Close relationships/friendships _____	Close relationships/friendships _____
Communication skills _____	Communication skills _____
Overall happiness _____	Overall happiness _____
Relationship with God _____	Relationship with God _____

As you answered the preceding questions, did you find any areas of your life that need adjustment? If so, accept God's grace and guidance as you look toward your desired destination.

Facing the Facts

The next step is especially relevant as we define your child's physical starting point. Talking about weight is never easy, and this discomfort intensifies when our beloved children are the focus of the discussion. In fact, as hot a topic as childhood obesity is right now, one of the hardest parts of dealing with an overweight child is acknowledging the truth: "My child is overweight." It isn't nearly as hard to say, "My child has asthma" or "My child isn't very good in math." But asthma and math don't pack the same emotional punch in our society as being overweight. As we face the truth, we may be haunted by many questions: *Is it my fault? Am I being too critical? Do kids make fun of him? Does she have a future?* When attempting to determine the appropriate size for your child, it may be extremely painful to admit the truth. And yet, *knowing* truth is the first step to *being set free.*

Consider this: If your child is overweight, he probably knows it. His friends or the mirror have already told him. But he may be dealing with it all alone if everyone else keeps avoiding the subject.

To obtain an accurate picture of your child's starting point, let's roll up our sleeves, gather up our courage and determine whether your child is obese, overweight or currently at her appropriate size. Once you know where you *are,* you can accurately plan your course on this life-changing journey.

Defining Childhood Obesity

Children always keep us guessing. Whether we're talking about their intel-
lectual development, physical growth or emotional maturity, children
rarely make steady, predictable progress. Rather, their development may
be characterized by long periods of little change interrupted by seasons of
radical change. Some parents worry about their 20-month-old son's limited vocabulary, only to witness him suddenly speaking in full sentences.
Changes in weight and growth are no exception, so developing a standard for the appropriate size for children isn't easy. Due to these uneven
growth spurts, it is hard to determine what is an appropriate weight just
by looking—especially if we don't really want to see the truth!

Currently, the most useful tool for an initial assessment of a child's
weight is based on the body mass index (BMI). The BMI takes into
account the normal differences in body fat between boys and girls, as
well as the amount of fat present at different ages. It is easy to calculate,
has national standards available for comparison and is extremely reliable. For these reasons, the Centers for Disease Control (CDC) and the
American Academy of Pediatrics (AAP) recommend the use of BMI to
screen for appropriate weights in children and teens.[3]

The BMI gives us a measurable index of the child's weight, which can
then be compared to that of all children of the same age and sex in order
to develop a BMI percentile. Many parents are familiar with percentiles
because they are used to describe height and weight beginning in infancy.
Higher percentiles mean the child is larger than other children of the same
age and sex, while lower percentiles mean he is smaller. However, no
method is completely foolproof, and so rare exceptions do occur. An adolescent who participates in body-building and has exceptional muscle mass
might have an abnormally high BMI, even though he isn't overweight. In
reality, though, most normal variations of activity and muscle mass do *not*
affect the reliability of the BMI. So, if your child has a high BMI, it is likely
that he is overweight. If you think your child may be an exception, perhaps
due to participation in an intense athletics program, you may wish to
speak with your pediatrician or family practitioner about it.

In defining childhood obesity, the words we use are important. If we
are to understand each other, we need to speak the same language! We will

use the specific terminology the CDC has developed for categorizing the weight of children. Based on their BMI percentile, children are described as "underweight," "at a healthy weight," "overweight" or "obese."

Most children's physicians calculate a child's BMI percentile at each preventive medicine visit, so it's likely that your child's doctor can provide you with his most recent report. Your child's BMI percentile can also be determined at different websites, by using standardized charts or based on a mathematic formula (refer to the appendix for instructions on how to determine your child's body mass index, BMI percentile and CDC weight category).

Keep in mind that the BMI is considered a screening tool rather than a diagnosis. Other components to help assess your child's health might include a physical examination, family history, activity level and additional screening tests. If your child is overweight or obese, then changes are needed.

Jennifer tells of her youngest child: "When my daughter gained weight as a youngster, I didn't even give it a second thought, knowing that kids can often go through a 'chunky' stage, just as her older sister had. However, as time passed, she *didn't* slim down, and in fact continued to *gain* weight! I wish I had taken notice sooner."

What Jennifer discovered is that, in today's culture, children in the "overweight" and "obese" categories are unlikely to achieve a normal weight on their own. So, it's important to sit up and take notice now, when simple and subtle changes can have transforming results.

If your child is *not* overweight, then you can focus on encouraging behaviors that will maintain optimum health.

If your child is underweight, then you may want to speak with your child's pediatrician.

Change of Perspective

Reflecting again on family vacations, you may feel that calculating your child's BMI and BMI percentile is much like spending all day studying a national monument in the blazing hot sun! You may be feeling restless and bogged down. If so, then it is time to change perspectives.

Those of you who are familiar with the *Thin Within* book and ministry may feel that weighing and measuring the height of your child in order to calculate the BMI represents a departure from our past philosophy. Rest assured this is not the case. Consider this passage from *Thin Within*, which is written to adults:

> We would like to encourage you to put the [bathroom] scale in its proper place . . . The scale can be used prayerfully, from time to time as a "reality check." We often think things are better or worse than they actually are. So using the scales as a reality check from time to time is okay.[4]

As adults, we have a good sense of an appropriate size and weight, and so we caution against frequent use of the scale because it can become a habit that is misused and abused. Still, on occasion it can provide a reality check as you make progress toward your natural, God-intended size.

In much the same way, calculating your child's BMI can be a useful tool as you seek to help your child achieve a healthy weight. While we adults tend to obsess over our weight, we may try to deny our child's weight problem, hoping to avoid facing the sad reality that she is not where she needs to be. Monitoring our child's BMI on occasion can keep us grounded in reality—and focused on leading our child toward better health and an appropriate weight. Remember, however, that your child is *not defined* by her BMI, any more than she is defined by her IQ.

Kim's mom obsessed about Kim's weight for much of her childhood, weighing her frequently and keeping her on a restrictive diet. Unfortunately, this process led Kim to believe that the bathroom scale was the ultimate measuring stick that defined her worth as a person. As an adult, her self-worth seems to ebb and flow based on her size. Accepting the unconditional love offered by God and her family remains a daily struggle.

In contrast to the approach used by Kim's mother, we recognize that physical size is only a part of the picture. Avoid allowing this tool to take on undue importance by frequently weighing your child or plotting dots on the BMI chart. We encourage you to utilize the BMI tool to help determine your starting point—and as an *occasional* measure of progress.

Medical Moment: The Big Picture

Every few years, a new national health survey is done. In recent decades, each new survey has indicated that American children are getting larger. From 1963 to 2002, the number of overweight children aged 6 to 19 *quadrupled*. Children who are overweight or obese now represent 30 percent of those aged 6 to 19, and 20 percent of 2- to 5-year-olds.[5] A recent study indicates that a significant percentage of young children *exceed the weight maximum for their car seat*, with few, if any, appropriate alternatives.[6] Is it any wonder that there seem to be overweight children wherever we turn?

The widespread impact of such a change is overwhelming. Cardio-vascular disease is being manifested at younger and younger ages, and Type 2 diabetes is now seen in children as young as 6 years of age. Other problems include fatty liver, gallstones, sleep apnea, and bone and joint problems.[7] In addition, overweight children suffer from low self-esteem and social isolation, and are at higher risk for psychological disorders such as depression and oppositional-defiant disorder.[8]

The sharp rise in childhood obesity has been accurately termed an epidemic and requires our full attention. While the statistics are scary, it isn't profitable to panic. Instead, it is time to accept the reality of what you are facing, commit your family to making some necessary changes and see what marvelous things God has in store for your child.

No matter what you discovered today, you have just won a big victory. Regardless of your family's starting point, and whatever your child's current BMI, celebrate the fact that *you can do something about it.* We ask that you accept your child's starting point as "science sense," but that you utilize "God's sense" to place it in proper perspective. Consider the words of 1 Samuel: "God does not see the same way people see. People look at the outside of a person, but the Lord looks at the heart" (16:7, *NCV*). As we move forward, hold on to that truth for dear life, and refuse to let it go.

Spirit Moment: Unconditional Love

As you reflect on your child's size, recognize that what he most needs from you is your unconditional love. Regardless of his weight or BMI calculations, he needs to know that you believe in *him*, not in what he can do or should do. So rather than exhibiting criticism, anxiety and frustration, keep a sense of optimism and compassion. While you may feel frustrated or fearful, remember that hope is on the way.

As you talk to your child about the need for changes, speak the truth in love (see Eph. 4:15). As you consider the daunting responsibilities you face and recall all of your accomplishments as a parent so far, remember that your ability to love stands at the top of the list. Love is certainly at the top of God's list when it comes to what is most important in life:

> If I speak with human eloquence and angelic ecstasy but don't love, I'm nothing but the creaking of a rusty gate. If I speak God's Word with power, revealing all his mysteries and making everything plain as day, and if I have faith that says to a mountain, "Jump," and it jumps, but I don't love, I'm nothing. If I give everything I own to the poor and even go to the stake to be burned as a martyr, but I don't love, I've gotten nowhere. So, no matter what I say, what I believe, and what I do, I'm bankrupt without love. Love never gives up. Love cares more for others than for self. Love doesn't want what it doesn't have. Love doesn't strut, doesn't have a swelled head, doesn't force itself on others, isn't always "me first," doesn't fly off the handle, doesn't keep score of the sins of others, doesn't revel when others grovel, takes pleasure in the flowering of truth, puts up with anything, trusts God always, always looks for the best, never looks back, but keeps going to the end. Love never dies (1 Cor. 13:1-8, *THE MESSAGE*).

Reading those words can be inspiring as well as overwhelming. Who of us can live up to all that? And yet, God is our ever-present help—He takes our feeble efforts and turns them into something beautiful. As you seek God's perfect love, you will find a renewed appreciation for your child. God chose you, with all your imperfections, to teach, motivate and care for your child. Trust Him and focus on loving your child every moment of every single day.

Every journey is marked by peaks and valleys, days of bright sunshine and dark, rainy nights. This one will be no different. As you face the challenges ahead with love, determination and commitment, take comfort from these words: You and your child are watched over by the One who cares for you more than you can imagine, and you are now on the right track.

Lord, we come to You with heavy, tender hearts for our children.
Please give us Your wisdom, and comfort us with the knowledge
that You are in control and that we can trust You to increase our faith
as You provide the answers we have been seeking.
Prepare our minds to learn, our ears to hear, and our hearts to love.
Thank You for Your steadfast love for each and every child,
and help us as parents to experience that love anew each day
as we travel this path.
Amen.

"For I know the plans I have for you," declares the LORD,
"plans to prosper you and not to harm you,
plans to give you hope and a future."
JEREMIAH 29:11

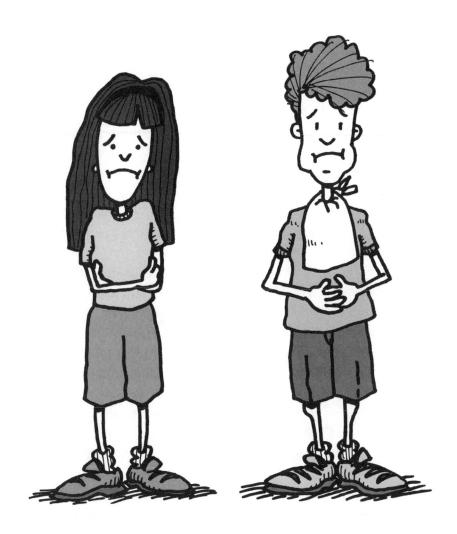

CHAPTER 3

HUNGER AND FULLNESS

When to Start and Stop Eating

It's rush hour on the freeway and Mom's "taxi service" is shuttling children from ballet practice to a basketball game. Bickering breaks out in the back seat and nerves wear thin. Desperate to restore calm, Mom is relieved to see hope on the horizon as the Golden Arches come into view! She exits the highway and plunges into the fast-food drive-thru lane. From the back seat comes a resounding, overjoyed "Yea!" Our heroine soon merges back onto the freeway, thinking, *They don't call them "Happy Meals" for nothing!* But was this *true* hunger? Not even close! *Survival mechanism?* You got it!

Can you relate to this scenario? The truth is, food is often used to celebrate a good day at school or to keep children quiet. Our reasons for eating often have *nothing* to do with true physiological hunger.

A recent family gathering captured a prevailing cultural value when Eric called his young son to the dinner table: "Jimmy, it's time to eat." His son, busily playing, responded, "But, Dad, I'm not hungry!" A near-by uncle laughingly responded, "What's *that* got to do with eating?"

It isn't easy to get a grip on hunger, satisfaction and fullness while living in America, the land of plenty. One mother shared about a time when her teenaged daughter was lamenting her brother's foul mood: "Daniela turned to me and said, 'Mom, *please* make some brownies for Mark so he'll be in a better mood!' Instantly I realized the poor example I'd set for my children in leading them to believe that food—more specifically, chocolate—can change a bad mood into a good one!"

There is often a disconnect between what we *physically need* and what we *actually eat*. The result is an obsession with bigger portions, endless choices, richer desserts and 24-hour availability. In a recent assault on our sensibilities, one fast-food chain advertised a "fourth meal"—as if three mega-portions aren't enough!

Life in America has moved into the "fast lane," and with it, the amount of food consumed is completely out of control. Portion sizes have sky-rocketed in the past 40 years. Cookies now exceed USDA standards by a whopping 700 percent and cooked pasta by 480 percent.[1] Some restaurant entrées can feed a family of four! Studies show that increased portion size results in overeating—without people realizing it.[2] Our children are being impacted by larger, less-healthy school lunches (check your local school's à la carte menu) and by bigger kids' meals in restaurants. A rippling effect of this phenomenon is that we are unconsciously increasing portion sizes at home because excessiveness has become the norm. As America has super-sized our food, our bodies have become super-sized, as well.

In the midst of this crazy food crisis, you might feel completely under-qualified to deal with your family's eating habits and your child's weight issues. But that's why we are here! Through practical, time-tested strategies, your entire family *can* learn to eat when hungry and stop when satisfied. Supporting and encouraging one another will not only help those who need to slim down but will also help leaner family members maintain their appropriate size and good health. It's a win-win situation, so stay the course!

Consider babies who intuitively know when to eat—and when not to—even if they don't have the words to express it. Pam shares the new eating strategies she learned by watching her toddler: "Allison was my example of a 'thin eater.' When she was hungry, I'd give her a banana, one of her favorite foods. After eagerly eating about half of it, she would slow down, and then suddenly drop the other half and go off to play. It was amazing to watch her *do* what I knew I *needed* to do." By following her internal cues of hunger, not only did this toddler grow into a healthy and fit young lady, but she also helped her mother lose 100 extra pounds!

At the age of eight, Pam's son Neil realized he was a bit pudgy and wanted to slim down. Pam shares his story with us:

> I told him about hunger and satisfaction, and shared how the Holy Spirit strengthened me and gave me the ability to wait for hunger and not eat beyond what my body needed. He began to follow my example and released 20 pounds over several months. I was so proud of him as he realized that overeating was not healthy or honoring to God.

To help you understand the concepts of hunger and satisfaction, we will explore two models. The first is that of an infant and the second is that of a naturally thin adult. As you examine these models, you will gain a new appreciation of God's miraculous design for your body, and the confidence that this is something that *you and your child can do.*

Model #1: The Infant

Most babies are perfect role models for appropriate eating habits—so we are going to learn from them for a change. Consider this: If an infant is hungry, he first begins to smack his lips, then he chews on his hand and finally fusses a bit. We all know what comes next: a loud, persistent cry! When the baby first senses hunger, he tries to soothe himself and then, when he's certain that he is *really* hungry, he tells the world! While we aren't advocating that we all scream for our supper, learning to test our hunger cues is a good habit to emulate.

Now consider the *amount* of food an infant eats. It's almost never the same from one meal to the next. A baby might breastfeed 15 minutes in the morning and twice as long in the afternoon, or drink four ounces at a single feeding and only two at the next. Why is that? *Because babies stop eating when satisfied.* Try to get her to eat more and you'll likely pay for it dearly—when she spits up all over the place!

Anyone with an overweight child can probably recall when his eating habits were just like this—self-regulated and healthy. In fact, you may have even been concerned at one point that he wasn't eating *enough.* Rest assured that you aren't the only one who has difficulty understanding how such a drastic change can occur. The good news is that while adults may have had bad eating habits for decades, children aren't so far removed from "doing it right." This means that your overweight child can recover those God-given instincts more quickly than you might imagine. When it comes to eating, "acting like a baby" might not be such a bad thing!

Model #2: The Naturally Thin Adult

Our next model, the naturally thin adult, is a person of great mystery in our food-focused culture. These folks have been naturally slender all their lives, seemingly without any effort. They don't diet; they aren't exercise junkies; they appear to eat whatever and whenever they want, and yet they are sized "just right." We may hold these people in awe—and may secretly hope they have at least *one* hidden character flaw!

For Andrea, eating is an enjoyable but somewhat incidental part of life. She typically eats small amounts of whatever is being served, without worrying about the calorie content. While she delights in the smell, appearance and taste of foods of all kinds (from decadent desserts to exotic salads), the best part of her meal is the shared fellowship. She eats slowly and methodically, then stops at a place of satisfaction before she is full. Andrea takes great pleasure in eating within wise boundaries and does so naturally. She enjoys being active and doesn't even own a bathroom scale. At 57 years of age, she continues to be the size she was when she was 17—without dieting!

This picture of a naturally thin person gives insight into how God created our bodies to respond to hunger, satisfaction and fullness. Rather than begrudging the naturally thin adult, let's learn from her and discover how to recapture our long-lost (but not entirely forgotten) hunger and satisfaction signals.

Now contrast the "naturally thin" style of eating with the behavior of most people you know. After commenting on how they feel stuffed, many take second or even third helpings. What about table conversation? While the naturally thin adult chatters away, oblivious to her food, others inhale their cheesecake as though it was their last meal. And how likely are most of us to *forget* to eat? Impossible! These behaviors show a stark contrast between the naturally thin individual who acknowledges and obeys the instincts of her body, and a person who does not. Unfortunately, many more Americans fall into the latter category than the former, and our children are learning all too quickly to follow in our super-sized footsteps.

So often we think we have to go to extremes to correct unworkable behavior, but it's important *not* to put our kids on a radical diet. Instead, our task is to use the models of the infant and the naturally thin adult to teach our children how God intended for us to relate to food and eating. In the process they will learn to eat the *right amount* of food—what their body truly needs—which is the first and most important step toward becoming a trim, fit kid.

Consider the following scenario of one family, long accustomed to concluding meals with a sugary dessert. When 13-year-old Leslie requested a cookie after lunch, her father asked, "Are you still hungry?"

Baffled, Leslie replied, "No, I didn't even finish my sandwich."

Her wise father said, "Yes, you may have a cookie—*when you are hungry again.*" Initially, this perplexed Leslie, but she accepted her father's answer because she knew a cookie would be waiting for her when she got hungry. In time, the family incorporated other options, such as fruit and yogurt, and gradually eliminated this "automatic" dispensing of sweets at the end of every meal.

What Went Wrong?

Infants, babies and most young children know when to start and stop eating. But gradually, the picky toddler may learn to "pig-out." Many factors can influence our God-given signals of hunger and satisfaction: friends, family, TV commercials, magazine ads, role models, teachers, and hectic schedules, to name a few. Sometimes these messages are healthy, but often they are not. As children begin to grow and stretch their wings, it is crucial that parents continue to provide appropriate guidance and structure when it comes to nutrition and physical fitness.

Getting the Point Across: The Balloon and Belly Meter

Now let's roll up our sleeves and get to work! The first task will be for your child to understand the concepts of an *empty* stomach, a *satisfied* stomach, and a *full* (or *stuffed*) stomach. The goal is for her to wait for a completely empty stomach before eating and to stop *before* feeling too full. To illustrate, we will use two visuals: a balloon and a meter.

Imagine a brand-new, uninflated balloon. This represents an empty stomach. As the balloon is filled with air or water, it begins to enlarge. When it has stretched a bit and assumes a nice rounded shape about the size of your child's fist, this represents a satisfied stomach. As it continues to fill, it will stretch to the point of almost bursting. This is the image of a *full* (or *stuffed*) stomach. The desired goal is for your child to wait for true hunger (like the empty balloon) before eating, and to stop eating when his stomach is comfortable, long before it reaches the point of "I'm so full I'm about to pop." (Be sure to point out to your child that his stomach will never burst!)

Another visual is that of a meter or gauge. A completely empty stomach, which is true hunger, registers 0 on the meter. When the stomach is satisfied, or "just right," this is 5 on the meter. When the stomach reaches that "after Thanksgiving dinner, can't eat another bite" level of fullness, that is 10 on the meter. The goal for your child is to wait for 0 to begin eating and to stop eating at a comfortable 5.

As children eat from "empty" to "satisfied," they will attain and maintain their appropriate weight. If your child is overweight or obese, eating from 0 to 5 will allow her to slim down. Your child's body will tell her when extra nutrition is needed. In a growth spurt she will reach hunger more quickly because her body needs more fuel, and you may feel as if you're feeding a bottomless pit. On the other hand, if she isn't in a time of rapid growth, she may not be hungry even for three meals a day. These are natural variations in your child's nutritional needs as she grows and matures.

Depending on your child's age, you might discuss hunger and fullness using the above illustrations. Make it a fun and informative experience, perhaps by using yourself as an example. "Do you remember when I ate *six* pieces of pizza? This is what my stomach felt like!" Then proceed to blow up the balloon until it is large and stretched. Before breakfast you might ask your child to describe how his tummy feels, demonstrating with an uninflated balloon what an empty tummy, or a stomach at a 0, looks like. (*Warning:* Latex balloons are a choking hazard for children, so please use them for illustration purposes only and do not allow your children to play with them without adult supervision!)

During meals, each person can discuss whether her stomach feels "still empty," "just right" or whether it is starting to get "too crowded," or "full." And if you or your child needs to lie down or loosen a waistband, explain that this is a sign of a stomach that is *way* too full—"about to pop," or a 10 on the belly meter. By using words and descriptions that your child understands, you can take turns sharing "tummy readings."

When you note your child responding to her natural hunger and satis-faction cues—and eating less—it's time for applause and high-fives!

The Eight Tummy Keys

Our next task is to address your child's eating environment using what we call the Tummy Keys. These are practical tips that will enable your overweight child to *eat less food* by recognizing the "state" of his stomach. We're not advocating imposing strict calorie requirements; rather, we want you to teach your child to be attuned to feedback from his God-given body. As we discuss each of these keys, remember to be patient. Rome wasn't built in a day, and neither will sound and healthy eating habits! Persistence *will* pay off and your child will gradually learn to eat only the amount of food his body needs.

Throughout our discussion, keep this important point in mind: If your child is overweight, then she is eating more food than she needs given her current activity level. You may feel she eats "almost nothing" compared to her older sister who "ate twice as much" at the same age. The fact is, overweight or obese children need to eat less food and move their bodies more.

Key #1: Wait for an Empty Tummy

This key is the cornerstone for nearly everything else, so it's worth some effort to get it right. In order for your child to be a trim and fit kid, it is extremely important for him to wait for true hunger before eating. Kids who snack all day long—the popular habit of "grazing"—never experi-ence true hunger because they don't allow their stomach to return to its normal, empty state.

As parents, our responsibility is to offer food to our children when it is appropriate. Are we like the taxi-driving mom who veered into the fast-food drive-thru in order to soothe her children's unhap-piness? Or are we like Daniela who wanted to "cure" her brother's grouchiness with brownies? Do we tend to feed our loved ones when faced with a challenging situation, rather than seek a more suitable, nonfood-related solution? As parents, we must be mindful of our use of food so that we can avoid stuffing our child's body *and* feelings with food.

So what should you do when your overweight child says, "But I'm *huuuuu*ngry!" with that pitiful, petulant look in her eye, even though she ate only one hour ago? You might begin by evaluating what she ate for her last meal or snack. Some foods sustain better than others. If she had a bowl of sugary cereal for breakfast, she may feel empty much sooner than if she had had an egg, toast and a glass of orange juice. Also, assess her activity since she last ate, recognizing that if she has been particularly active, her body probably *does* require more fuel.

If you discern that your child's sensations may not be genuine hunger, then consider a distraction, such as playing together, to capture his interest and allow you to "test" his hunger. Also reassure him that an empty stomach is not harmful. Explain that as his tummy empties, his body will feel lighter and he will enjoy jumping and running more easily. It is perfectly healthy and acceptable for your child to experience the feeling of true hunger. The truth is, God-given hunger is good and very freeing. Be sure to teach him that he is unique—and is indeed God's wonderful masterpiece.

Restaurants can be opportune places to address hunger in a positive manner. When your children proclaim, "We're starving!" calmly respond, "Boy, I'm hungry, too. That means our food will taste great when we finally get to eat! Let's play a game until the food arrives." This teachable moment can help children understand that hunger isn't something to panic about. It's also an opportunity for them to develop patience by learning the art of delayed gratification.

Key #2: Bottoms Down!

So much of our eating is done on the run, dashing from place to place, driving the kids to swimming lessons or back and forth to school. This may seem like a convenient time-saver but, unfortunately, eating on the run isn't very satisfying and sets a poor example for our children. While multitasking is quite common in our fast-paced culture, we all need to *sit down* to eat—and eating while in the car *doesn't* count! This will allow your child to hear what his tummy has to say about hunger and satisfaction, while he sits down on his bottom, relaxes and enjoys connecting with his family.

Key #3: Press the Mute Button

Think about all the distractions that can occur during meals: TV, phone calls, radios . . . and family arguments! All too often, our food is consumed quickly and unconsciously. When we don't focus on our food, we forget about when we last ate. We may wonder aloud, "Did I eat breakfast?" Or if we've been distracted and failed to savor the eating experience, we may feel cheated and go back for seconds.

We highly recommend that at mealtime you pretend you have a huge "mute" button for everything other than dinner table conversation. Turn off the TV, ignore the phone and avoid other major distractions. We encourage your entire family to sit down together and focus only on the meal and each other. Call a truce on family disputes and sensitive issues. Don't be afraid to set mealtime rules designating the dinner table as a no-whining, no-fighting zone, and declaring the complaint department closed! Relish the food and personal interaction—period. This will enable each person to recognize clearly the stomach's "satisfied" signals and prevent overeating. As mealtimes become less chaotic and more peaceful, you'll be amazed at how enjoyable your eating experience can become.

Mealtimes in the Bible were considered sacred times of fellowship, love and worship. Explain to your child that meals are an important time for the entire family to connect, laugh together and demonstrate love for one another. It can provide an opportunity for each person to share about their day at school or work, the funny moment during piano lessons, or the new masterpiece completed in art class. Such shared memories will last a lifetime and are much more important than Monday night football or the latest celebrity scandal.

Key #4: Remember the Power of Prayer

Don't forget to give thanks for every meal. Prayer helps us to pause in the midst of our hectic day to focus our hearts and minds on the Lord. It helps us break out of the gobble-it-down mindset with which many of us approach mealtime, and sets an example of thankfulness that will follow our children into adulthood.

Before prayer, ask your children for any prayer requests, or ask your child to pray. Holding the hand of your child and hearing her talk to

God will help put everything in perspective! Thank God for the delightful flavors, smells and appearance of the food He has graciously provided. Pray for discernment for all family members so that they might stop eating when they are satisfied. Teach your child that having plentiful food and a loving family are blessings from God that are to be savored and appreciated.

Key #5: Slow Down!

A lady was pulled over for speeding and the policeman asked, "Didn't you see the speed limit sign?" She replied truthfully, "No, officer, I was going too fast to read it!" Just as you can't read a road sign when speeding, your child can't listen to feedback from his tummy if he's stuffing the food in too quickly. The most common reason for eating past the point of satisfaction is eating too fast. Before you sit down to your next family meal, let everyone know that the new plan is to slow down. Explain that this gives everyone the chance to enjoy their food, as well as to check in with their tummies so that they will know when they are satisfied.

Once you've laid out the new game plan, the best thing you can do is model the following strategies:

1. Put the fork or spoon down between each bite.

2. Chew each bite completely and swallow it before shoveling in another forkful of food. You might explain that the mouth doesn't enjoy being "too crowded." Besides, a huge mouthful of food is not a pretty sight!

3. Finish chewing and swallowing food before drinking a beverage. Washing food down often diminishes flavor and enjoyment and may lead to a craving for more food.

One last piece of advice here: Avoid becoming a nag. If your child is still wolfing down her food, respectfully instruct her without commands or demands. Otherwise, your good intentions can cause emotional outbursts that create even more tension. You might consider this approach: "Boy, this chicken enchilada is so good; I'm tempted to eat it *too* fast! But I'm going to slow down so I can really enjoy every bite! Can you help me remember to slow down a little?" We can't emphasize enough that your example speaks volumes.

Key #6: Eat Yummy Food!

This key doesn't mean you should serve your family a bowl of M&Ms for dinner. And yet, one huge mistake parents often make is to insist that children eat food they really don't like and then withhold foods they enjoy. Forcing an unwanted food on your children often makes things worse. All too often, parents may decide that their children are going to eat a particular food "because I said so!" Once that happens, the battle is no longer about nutrition but about power.

Kathy's childhood experiences created issues that she continues to deal with even today. "I have vivid memories of knock-down, drag-out fights in which my parents literally forced food into my mouth. I was told that the green peas I didn't eat at dinner would be served to me again—cold—at every meal until I finally gave in and ate them. My parents were convinced that if I were hungry enough, I would learn to like those cold, shriveled peas. But they were wrong! I became a horrible sneak, swiping money to buy candy bars, just so I wouldn't be hungry. As a result of the pressure, I developed a gag reflex every time I tried to eat vegetables. To this day I *still* can't cope with green peas."

Kathy's story demonstrates that when the dinner table becomes a battleground, everyone loses. To avoid battles over food, consider this practical advice.

First, remember that children's portion sizes should be much smaller than you think. A serving size of peas for a toddler is about a teaspoon. So the "three bites" of a food your daughter won't eat could mean you've exceeded the serving size! Would you like to eat a full portion (or more) of something you hate? Probably not. Instead, ask her to taste a tiny bit on the end of the spoon or on the tip of her finger and leave it at that. Kirsten, a mother of three naturally thin children, calls this the "no, thank you" bite. After your child tastes just a small amount on several occasions, she either *will* or *won't* develop a taste for it. If she still doesn't like the food, then accept it and let it go! Perhaps you can try it again when she's a bit older.

Another common parenting concern is that a "picky" child will miss out on important nutrients or vitamins. While this concern is understandable, consider the fact that millions of young children go through a picky stage in their development, and yet malnutrition in this country is extremely rare. On the other hand, obesity is increasing every day. Please don't let your fear of an unbalanced diet lead you to force-feed or overfeed your child. The risk of obesity is greater than the risk of malnutrition, and most picky eaters ultimately wind up eating a well-balanced diet over the long haul. If you are really concerned about vitamins and nutrition, ask your doctor if he or she would recommend a once-a-day vitamin for your child.

What about desserts? Some really strange rationales are often used when it comes to whether or not a child can have dessert. Mandy describes her frustration over her grandmother's "clean your plate" rule. "At breakfast I love strawberries with sugar sprinkled on top. But I can't have them unless I first eat my eggs, two pieces of bacon and a biscuit. By the time I eat all that, I'm stuffed!"

While most of us aren't comfortable allowing our children to refuse food on their plate and then eat a big bowl of ice cream, please don't tell your child that he has to "clean his plate" before he can have dessert. This does two things, neither of which is helpful. First, it makes dessert even more attractive, because you are using it as a reward. Second, you are inadvertently teaching him to overeat. By the time he finishes everything you have required him to eat, he will be satisfied. But you promised him dessert, so, by golly, he's going to eat it whether he's hungry or not!

What's a better solution? Consider having dessert only at some meals. Or perhaps use dessert occasionally as a replacement for a snack or meal when your child is truly hungry.

Lastly, although it's a good idea to keep your child's preferences in mind when preparing meals, don't be a short-order cook. Why? Because your child will quickly figure out how to get you to serve only the foods she likes (when she wants them), and she won't be motivated to try other foods. Of course, if she doesn't like what's served, she may pick at it or skip it entirely—and that's okay. She'll be even hungrier at the next meal, and food that wasn't her first choice may become more appealing. Remember, eating less food is good, not bad.

God created us to gravitate toward the things we like in all areas of life. But some really good things take time to appreciate. Many of the things we enjoy as adults—good music, a peaceful walk, art, gardening, reading—were probably not favorites in our childhood years. And had they been forced on us in a heavy-handed manner, our interest would not have been cultivated any sooner and perhaps not at all. This applies to good food as well. Be patient and provide your child with a variety of nutritious and pleasing food options, then let him decide what and how much to eat.

Don't be afraid to be a kid again yourself. If you are willing to revisit your taste for cotton candy, maybe your child will be willing to try a bite of shitake mushroom! When your child genuinely chooses a nutritious food, then celebrate! You have given her a gift that will last forever.

Key #7: Manners Matter

Table manners are all about courtesy and good sense. "Don't talk with your mouth full." "Swallow your food before drinking." In addition to teaching respect and courtesy, good manners can also encourage healthy eating habits. So begin teaching your child these lessons when he is very young. When someone else is talking, it's respectful for him to lay down his eating utensils, look at the person and listen to what she is saying. When your child wants to talk, he should avoid interrupting, and he should finish talking before resuming eating or drinking. If your child is still young enough to need hands-on guidance, sit next to him and, when he begins talking, you can gently take his hand and place it on the table so that he remembers not to eat and talk at the same time. In the process, the whole family will learn to eat more slowly, enjoy each other's company and pay more attention to the food.

This can also be a great time for teaching some "life lessons" such as respect, humility, self-control and patience. The entire family will be practicing these character qualities together, remembering that actions always speak louder than words.

Key #8: Don't Pop . . . Learn When to Stop!

As pointed out earlier, most babies and very young children instinctively know to eat when truly hungry and to stop eating when satisfied. But older children and adults are often greatly influenced by our super-sized culture and may not recognize when to stop eating. Because it takes 20 to 30 minutes for the brain to register just how full the stomach is, you can easily eat beyond the point of satisfaction. For this reason, talk to your child about how her tummy feels at the start of the meal, in the middle, at the end and then a half-hour after the meal. If she feels really full after eating, just say, "Wow, your tummy must have gotten too crowded. Next time, let's try to remember to stop eating a little sooner."

Avoid controlling, condemning or shaming, but rather use wisdom as you apply these principles. You will be building your relationship with your child instead of tearing it down. Childhood obesity is a crisis for many, but God can use it to strengthen the bonds within your family as each person commits to being as healthy and fit as possible.

Do everything you can to minimize temptations to eat inappropriately in your home. Avoid putting extra bowls of food on the dining table—leave them in the kitchen so that your table is cleared of all clutter, except for decorative items such as candles or flowers. Decrease portions by serving food on smaller plates (such as salad plates), cook less food or put the excess in the freezer so that second helpings aren't an option. Remember: *If your child is overweight, he is eating more food than he needs given his current activity level.*

Common Sense Corner

Many parents are stumped by how to implement guidelines regarding food and eating. The most practical parent who manages to keep three kids, a dog and a cat in line may suddenly become tongue-tied when talking with her child about food. There seems to be an inherent fear among parents that *any* boundary setting—at least when it comes to food—may cause lifelong damage to our children.

Yet it's our job as parents to create boundaries for our children, so follow the same parenting principles that work in other areas. Set clear boundaries, give reasonable explanations and leave it at that. If you offer to buy your child a toy, how would you respond if he demanded two or three? Most likely you would say, "One is enough" without giving it a second thought. Yet when a similar scenario presents itself when it comes to food, you might be concerned that saying no to a second helping might be inappropriate. This fear may stem from your own issues, so try to recognize this when it's time to set wise food limits for your children. Your child will respect the boundaries and will *not* be emotionally scarred by the experience.

As you reflect on the tools we have discussed in this chapter, you may feel as though your brain is overloaded. If so, go easy on yourself. Some of these concepts may be brand-new and may take some time to sink in.

We believe it is helpful to keep track of your progress, so we have included a chart in the appendix to help you and your child record how well the Tummy Keys are being followed. In addition, a journal might be helpful so that you can record your thoughts, ideas or inspirations on your journey toward healthy living—for your child and yourself.

In the next chapter we will address hunger and satisfaction as they apply to specific ages and stages of development. As you progress on your journey of raising a child who is fit on the inside as well as the outside, continue to look to the Lord for moment-by-moment guidance.

Lord, our family needs to implement many changes
as we seek to live out a new approach to food and eating.
Please provide the strength to do what is necessary
as we seek the path that You desire for us.
We pray that You will guide and direct us every step of the way.
Make us a team looking to You, Lord, so that we all can
move toward a life that is pleasing to You in every way.
Thank You so much for Your patience and unconditional love.
Amen.

Trust God from the bottom of your heart; don't try to figure out everything on your own. Listen for God's voice in everything you do, everywhere you go; he's the one who will keep you on track.

PROVERBS 3:5-6, *THE MESSAGE*

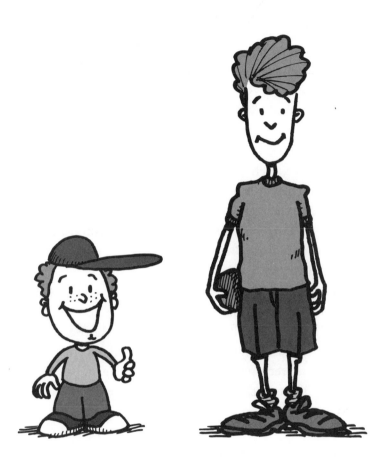

CHAPTER 4

AGES AND STAGES

Practical Hunger and Fullness Tips

L et the roller-coaster ride begin!" Chances are, in the excitement of the moment, you don't remember the exact words that were spoken when that cuddly bundle was first placed in your eager arms. But one thing is for sure: The serene, innocent face of your newborn gave you absolutely no hint of the radical changes that lay ahead!

From the sleepless nights of infancy through the complete mystery of adolescence, each age and stage brings its own joys and challenges. No doubt about it, kids turn our lives upside down! And yet, we wouldn't trade them for anything in the world. Regardless of what challenge you are currently facing, consider this: Almost *every* parent with grownup kids wishes they had enjoyed their children a little more and worried a little less.

The various ages and stages that your child goes through call for an assortment of practical tools. In this chapter, you will find many suggestions that apply specifically to your child's current age, but feel free to glean helpful insights from reading all the tips. Becoming familiar with our recommendations for all the stages of development may shed light on the past and help you prepare for a more successful future.

And one last word before you dig in: Our insights are meant to be utilized *alongside* your parental instincts. Remember, you know your child better than anyone else!

Infancy (Birth to One Year)

If your child hasn't celebrated her first birthday yet, then your focus will be on developing good habits right from the start. The good news is that the weight of babies under a year of age does not correlate with later obesity, so please don't worry at this point about weight or BMI. However, the development of poor eating habits at this stage *can* significantly increase the risk of being overweight later on. By establishing fit kid habits now, your child can avoid becoming a childhood obesity statistic! The tips we share here will enable you to avoid the common pitfalls that are prevalent in our culture today.

Medical Moment: Breastfeeding Versus Bottle Feeding

Whether you are a new mom or feel that you are over the hill, breast-feeding remains an important issue. Few areas generate more debate and anxiety, and even mothers of teenagers may have remnants of smugness or guilt depending on whether they chose—*15 years ago*—to feed by breast or bottle! We are sensitive to the personal nature of this issue and want to reassure you that we have no intention of telling you what to do or of criticizing a prior decision you may have made. Instead, using all our "senses," we will discuss the medical and emotional aspects of the topic. You will then be equipped to make your own decision regarding the future—or to appropriately, not emotionally, evaluate the impact of past decisions.

Because of many nutritional benefits of breast milk, breastfeeding is recommended by the American Academy of Pediatrics for children up to one year of age (of course, after the child is a year old, the appropriate time for weaning is up to Mom and baby). Breastfed infants may be less likely to develop bacterial meningitis, ear infections, sudden infant death syndrome (SIDS), types 1 and 2 diabetes, leukemia, obesity, asthma, and many other medical problems. Beyond that, as a group, breast-fed babies show slightly higher performance on cognitive IQ tests.[1] Sounds pretty wonderful, doesn't it? Since God has designed such a super, ready-made nutrient, it is prudent for every new mom to make an educated decision regarding how she will nourish her newborn.

Babies aren't the only ones who benefit from breastfeeding. Mothers benefit as well, with less postpartum bleeding, earlier return to pre-partum weight, decreased risk of breast and ovarian cancer, and possibly decreased osteoporosis.[2] Equally important is the bonding that occurs during breastfeeding, giving both mother and baby a sense of security and fulfillment that is difficult to explain, measure or duplicate.

Despite its merits, breastfeeding, at times, is not always the clear choice. Some women are too scared to give it a try, while others have every intention of breastfeeding but something prevents it from happening. Some families simply want Dad more involved in feeding right from the start. Sadly, women who don't breastfeed for whatever reason are often made to feel guilty by others. Between postpartum hormones and the stress of a newborn infant, the *last* thing a new mom needs is added insecurity!

If you are struggling with this decision, consider the nutritional and medical advantages (science sense), as well as your own unique situation (common sense). Consider speaking with a pediatrician or a lactation consultant for added confidence and direction. Utilize "God's sense" as you prayerfully seek His guidance. Finally, make an informed decision and stick to it.

Regardless of your decision, please recognize that breastfeeding *isn't* a "line in the sand" separating the good from the bad. Many infants are appropriately nourished by infant formula. If you are unable to breast-feed for medical or personal reasons, you will have ample opportunity to bond with your child and to help him learn to be attuned to his God-given instincts and develop wonderful eating habits. Whether nursing or bottle-feeding, your most important job is to follow your infant's cues of hunger and satisfaction, savoring this precious miracle from God.

Some Additional Tips for Infants

Now that we've made it through the tricky debate about infant feeding, let's move on to some tips that will apply to all infants, whether breast- or bottle-fed.

Don't Count Ounces!

Obeying natural hunger and fullness signals will almost always result in an infant's eating varying amounts at each meal. So, if your child is eating the same amount at every feeding, you may be "pushing" beyond her natural satisfaction signals without realizing it. If necessary, black out the ounce indicators on the bottle with a permanent marker so that you won't be tempted to let those markers dictate how much you feed your baby. Even at this early stage, you want to teach your child to eat when hungry and stop when satisfied.

Make Sure It Is Hunger

When your baby begins to fuss, *do* respond immediately, but *don't* immediately assume that he is hungry. Sleep-deprived parents naturally conclude that if the baby is fussing, he *must* be hungry. To be certain it's "true" hunger, consider checking the following possibilities (and add some of your own) before you decide to feed your baby.

1. Physical comfort—As you've probably experienced, babies don't like to be hot, cold or wet, so tending to these needs is always the first order of business. Before assuming she is hungry, check to see if your baby feels sweaty or cool to the touch; then add or remove clothes accordingly. It's amazing how a change of clothes and a fresh diaper can transform tears to contentment!

2. Emotional needs—Young babies crave security and need constant reminders that they are loved and cared for. You cannot spoil young infants by responding too quickly to their cries. In fact, the opposite is true: Infants who develop a secure, loving bond with their parents at an early age are better behaved and cry less as they get older.[3]

   If your baby simply needs your attention, then he will respond to cuddling, snuggling, humming or singing. Try different positions; some infants like to be snuggled on your body, others want to be facing outward, while still others prefer being held while you walk. As your baby gets older, continue to respond to his needs, but don't feel like you must jump the instant he makes a sound. Older babies are capable of entertaining themselves until you are able to pick them up, and they definitely do not always need to be fed at the first sign of being upset.

   Dorene shares about bringing her baby home after spending a traumatic week in the Neonatal Intensive Care Unit. "When Ruthie came home from the hospital, it seemed as if she wanted to nurse around the clock! My delight quickly gave way to exhaustion! She nursed and fussed, spit up and fussed some more. In hindsight, had I tried something other than feeding, we both would have been happier."

Ruthie was making up for lost time by seeking increased bonding time, but Dorene reacted as most of us would, mistakenly assuming Ruthie's discomfort was from hunger. When faced with a fussy infant, consider other possibilities before concluding that food is the answer. This will help your child be more comfortable and develop good eating habits. Remember that what works one time may not work the next time. Persevering through these challenges with your newborn is part of the high calling of parenting.

3. Boredom—Babies are born with thoughts, feelings and curiosity, but no way to get where they want or say what they need! To address possible boredom, consider changing rooms, go outside, move him to a swing or stationary walker (if old enough), or interact with him by playing next to him on the floor. As you develop creative ways to interact with your baby, you'll find the fussiness improves—for both of you!

4. Actions speak the loudest! Study your child and learn all about your precious gift from God. Once you understand, connect with and appreciate her uniqueness, it will ease the irritation when she gets cranky. As you respond with gentleness, you might find that simply speaking to your baby or rocking her gently will be enough to fend off fussiness. On the other hand, if you respond to your baby's cries with annoyance (which we all do from time to time), then nothing other than food will settle your child down. Why? Because your baby may decide that if she cannot get comfort from you, then she will get her comfort from food. As you can well imagine, even at a young age, this could set your child up for some eating issues that may be hard to overcome later.

Watch for Signs of Satisfaction
When your baby is eating (whether from the breast, bottle or spoon), pay very close attention to any sign that indicates he is losing interest.

If he is looking around, babbling or interested in something other than food, enjoy the moment and go with it! Please do not refocus him on the food. Instead, follow his cues, put the food aside and interact with him in whatever way he seems interested. Trying to get in a few more bites teaches him to eat past the point of satisfaction, which is a very difficult habit to break later on. You will want to protect and preserve the wonderful, natural, God-given instincts built into your baby. So if he remains disinterested, put the food away and declare the meal over!

In this area, breastfeeding gives us a good model to follow. When a breastfed infant begins to tire a bit, the suckling changes, and the milk flow slows down to a trickle. Bottles cannot duplicate that miraculous feat, so you need to watch closely for signs of tiring, and gently remove the bottle when they occur.

Introducing Solid Foods

Most experts recommend the introduction of solid foods to your infant when she is between four and six months of age, although breastfed infants may wait a little longer to begin solids. This timing allows babies to grow appropriately and develop the ability to manipulate textured foods in their mouths. Feeding your baby cereal or other baby foods too early can cause rapid weight gain (especially if she is getting solid foods in addition to her regular bottle or breastfeeding) and is also linked to development of food allergies.[4]

Introducing Table Foods

This new adventure is typically a time of immeasurable delight for both parent and child. While lots of fun, it is important to tread carefully, as it can be the beginning of a slippery downhill slide. While it is highly entertaining to see the expressions on a baby's face when she is fed different foods, babies should not be fed desserts and other rich foods—no matter how much fun Grandpa thinks it is! When introducing table foods, the content and consistency should be very similar to that of baby foods. Keep it simple, be a good role model, and don't give in to outside pressure from friends or family.

Be a Myth Buster

Resist buying into the myths that fat babies are healthier or that feeding your baby more than he needs will improve his disposition. Instead, follow your pediatrician's guidance regarding appropriate growth, and ask for help learning nonfood-related ways to improve sleep or deal with other behavior issues. If your baby remains very fussy or acts hungry all the time, then talk with your baby's doctor to make sure there isn't an underlying medical problem.

Prioritize!

Taking care of your baby is your most important job! In this day and age, young parents have a lot to juggle. Sheila tells of her experience as a new mom: "I needed to go shopping for groceries, but on the way out the door, I caught an unmistakable 'whiff' of a messy diaper, sending us back inside. After a fresh diaper and change of clothes, I successfully conquered buckling my baby in the back seat . . . then realized I had forgotten my wallet! I frantically ran back inside, located the wallet and made it back before my baby realized he had been abandoned. When I finally got the car started, I noticed my gas tank was almost empty! After stopping to fill up, I just felt exhausted and turned around and went back home."

Maybe you can identify with Sheila. In that moment, returning home was probably the best thing this stressed-out mom could do! The demands of motherhood can be overwhelming at times. In order to simplify life, whenever feasible, place your baby's needs above cleaning the house, catching up on paperwork or completing any other activities that you might feel are priorities. In 15 years, you will have forgotten how your house looked or whether you completed a job assignment to perfection, but you likely will recall the exact look on your baby's face when she took her first step. Give yourself permission to be fully present for those miraculous moments.

Toddlers and Preschoolers (Ages One to Four Years)

At this stage of the game, your gurgly baby has grown into an irresistibly cute, occasionally intimidating toddler who is equipped with an iron will and a striking resemblance to the Energizer bunny! Perhaps the following description by Erma Bombeck will strike a cord of familiarity:

> When I picked up the phone, like mechanical robots on schedule
> they gargled bleach, rolled potatoes across the floor, climbed on
> top of the TV set and took off all their clothes. When I said, "No,"
> they giggled; "Not now," they bit me; "Come to Mama," they ran
> into the traffic; "Let me see what is in your hand," they ate it;
> "The strained lamb is good for you," they blew it back in my face.
> Communicate with a toddler? I'd sooner take my chances with
> an untrained, excited puppy on a new white carpet.[5]

While your experience may be less dramatic, the fact remains that
the toddler years represent a unique stage! Your child's drastic personality shift, combined with a sudden change in his development, make
these years a challenging time to instill good eating habits. Although it
may be tempting to give up on proper nutrition during this stage, it is
important to realize that your child's size during this stage now begins
to have long-term impact. Further, your toddler is developing eating
habits that will last a lifetime. Remember, his eyes are on you, and he is
more likely to do what you do than what you say. So, dig in your heels
and let's attack those toddler issues.

Don't Panic Over a Poor Appetite

After the first year of life, your toddler's growth rate slows drastically.
If it didn't and she continued to grow at the same rate that she did in
the first year, she would one day be the size of a baby elephant! So, after
that first year, your child's food intake *needs* to decrease because there
isn't as much growth to support. If your child seems to turn up her
nose frequently at certain foods, we encourage you to go with the flow
and allow her cues for hunger and satisfaction to direct her eating and
your feeding.

Make Sure It's Hunger

Just because he has learned to say words that convey that he's "hungry,"
it doesn't necessarily mean his stomach is empty. Children respond to
non-verbal cues, so if you continue to address other needs first and

don't jump at his first announcement of hunger, he will learn that signs of hunger aren't cause for panic. If your toddler is overweight or obese, remember that he needs to eat less and move more. A good way to accomplish the former is by spacing out meal times and waiting for your child to experience true hunger before you feed him.

Self-Serve, Please

Allow your toddler to feed herself. By this stage, she is entirely capable of using her fingers or a spoon, and your assistance is not helpful. Decide on what her options will be (we will talk more about food choices in the next chapter), then let her decide how much to eat. You may not think she is eating enough, but she is as long as her growth is appropriate.

Recognize Satisfaction

When your child is no longer interested in what's on his plate, don't refocus him on the food—even if he has eaten only three bites. Your child will naturally grow less during this stage, so less food is required. Don't *ever* try to force-feed your toddler. You will always lose this kind of power struggle—and besides, you'll make a huge mess and his nutrition will not improve one bit! When your toddler throws the food on the floor, rather than trying to convince him to eat more, simply accept this as a not-so-subtle hint that he is finished and end the meal. You want eating to remain an emotionally pleasant experience, rather than a tension-filled event!

Make Meals Brief

During this stage, your toddler is less interested in eating but *very* interested in developing and practicing physical skills. Because of this, she will eat just enough to feel comfortable, then be ready to escape and practice her new climbing technique. Accept these God-designed tendencies, and set your toddler free!

All Done!

Hunger has been satisfied, and the meal is over. It is time to clean up, put the food away and get ready to do other things. However, a toddler can be very manipulative and love nothing more than to scream "down" while in the high chair, only to demand "eat" fewer than 10 minutes later. Calmly respond by saying, "We're all done eating for now, so let's find something to play together." Avoid arguing or pleading—once it gets emotional, the toddler always wins! Leave the kitchen, clean up the high chair, remove any bottles or plates that might remind your child of food, and move on. After following this pattern consistently, your child will understand that when a meal is over, it is really over.

Keep Food Out of Reach
Don't allow your toddler access to food between meals, even more nutritious choices like fruit. Constantly making food available will teach your child to "graze" all day long, rather than waiting for true hunger. As a result, he will begin to lose the ability to appreciate the stomach's signals regarding hunger and satisfaction. When it is time for a snack or a meal, place your toddler in a high chair and bring out the food. When his hunger has been satisfied, put the food away and send him on his way.

Let Eating Time Be for Eating
As you will see in other ages and stages, we advocate that when we feed our kids, that is all we do. The TV is turned off, and the telephone is either muted or ignored. However, pleasant music can be enjoyed if it is soothing and relaxing.

The School-Age Years (Ages Five Years and Above)

Just as you are ready to pat yourself on the back for surviving the toddler years, another challenge is coming down the pike. Remember those four-year-old snuggles, the sweet pats on your face, the dramatic hand motions and the feeling that you are the center of your child's universe? After beginning kindergarten, your sweet little child begins to mimic her friends, believe her teacher's opinion over your own and correct the words you use. And before you blink, your child is attending middle-school dances, requesting a cell phone and learning to drive. What on earth has happened? Well, God has designed for your child to . . . *sniff, sniff* . . . grow up. Consider this: If your children remained as adorable as at age four, we would never allow them to move out, and procreation would come to a screeching halt! So unless you want to be responsible for the end of the world, it's time to let go!

As you begin to release control over your child's environment and choices, your strategies regarding food will also require some flexibility and creativity. When your child begins to "own" eating according to hunger and satisfaction, you will begin to take on more of a coaching role. Walking the fine line between guidance and control is important, and your own behavior will be crucial. An adolescent who sees her dad eat only to meet his nutritional requirements is less likely to use food to numb her disappointment when she doesn't make the varsity basketball team.

(A note about adolescents: The eating habits of teenagers is a particularly difficult subject that could easily fill a volume all its own. Their habits range from those of a toddler to those of an adult, so we have chosen to include tips for younger adolescents in the section for children ages five years and above. Older adolescents may benefit from *Thin Within* by Judy and Arthur Halliday, a resource that is directed more toward adults.)

Make Family Meals a Priority

It is more important at this stage than any other to make meals a time of pleasant interaction for the entire family. Be forewarned: We must be intentional about this. Children at this stage develop a full social calendar, sweeping the family into a constant whirlwind of activities and commitments. Rather than grabbing meals on the run, allow enough time to sit down and eat, making fellowship the main event. In doing so, you will teach your child lifelong lessons about commitment, priorities and overall health. Your child will never forget the home-cooked meals and the love and meaningful interaction shared around the table.

As your children get older, you can help them "plan" their hunger to facilitate dining together. If dinner is served at 6 P.M., it helps if you can all *plan* to have an empty stomach at 6 P.M. For instance, if Julie gets hungry at 4 P.M. but wants to be "on empty" for the family meal at 6 P.M., her solution might be to have a few almonds or half an apple—just enough to fend off hunger until 6 P.M. rolls around. If Joey gets hungry at 5:15, he can either have a small cup of milk or remind himself that being hungry for 45 minutes won't mean the end of the world! These are some strategies your family can adopt in order to be able to have everyone arrive hungry at a planned dinner hour.

Less Is More

In today's culture, school-aged children who are obese are unlikely to slim down on their own without some guidance and intervention. If your child is overweight at this stage, eating less food by acknowledging hunger and fullness is an important first step in order to achieve his appropriate size. Talk with your child about the need to eat less, using non-emotional language appropriate for his maturity level. Develop reasonable boundaries and continue to work on hunger and satisfaction signals to decrease the quantity of food being consumed.

Be a Teacher

This is an important time of transition for you and your child. No longer can you childproof your home and guarantee your child's safety, but instead you must pray that you have successfully taught her how to keep herself safe when you aren't around. In the same way, you are in the process of teaching her how to eat from "0 to 5" without your hands-on support. Use your child's independence and interest in learning to your advantage, and prepare her for the temptations she will face when eating in social situations. Be informed about foods that are offered at school, and engage her in conversation about the food choices she makes when she's away from your watchful eye.

Heather recalls that as a young teenager, she began to gain weight—quickly. "During seventh grade, I moved from a small private school to a large public junior high. There was a great deal of stress at home and moving to a new school didn't help. My dad gave me money to buy lunch without realizing that food prices were much lower than he thought, so I actually had enough money to buy a *second* breakfast . . .

a huge, sticky cinnamon bun! Lunch was frequently a cheese and pepperoni pizza, followed by a cookie the size of a small Frisbee! My parents had no idea that what I ate at school was so nutritionally unsound. While they criticized me for being fat, it didn't occur to them that what I ate at school was a large part of the problem."

Being informed of the food options at school, club functions and friends' homes isn't always feasible, but if you have done your job, your child will begin to own "0 to 5" eating no matter where they are.

Our discussion of this topic would not be complete without addressing the difference between a "teacher" and a "controller." Many children resent their parents' nagging, controlling, criticizing or punishing them when it comes to their eating habits and nutrition and—you guessed it—they begin to sneak food! Your gut reaction to this might be to get angry or feel personally wronged by your child's dishonesty, but a more appropriate response is to ask if there is something going on that may be contributing to this behavior. We need to be aware that the environment we create, the relationships we foster and the humility (or lack of) with which we approach our children will affect their choices. Remember how Kathy (from chapter 3) responded to the radical measures her parents used to try to get her to eat peas? The last thing we as parents want to do is cause one of our own children to stumble.

Work on Words

As we mentioned earlier, when talking about eating habits and nutrition, practice using kind words that are age appropriate. Younger children might understand a tummy that feels "empty," "just right" or "too crowded." An older child might understand the idea of an "empty," "satisfied" or "full" stomach—or the concept of eating from "0 to 5." Offer examples of what might happen if his body gets too thin (feeling weak, not enough energy, not as strong)—or too heavy (unable to run as fast or jump as high, difficulty getting up from the floor or climbing stairs). Avoid saying, "You're going to get fat," "You'll never find a boyfriend" or other emotionally packed phrases. Comments such as these may scare your child and create anxiety rather than motivate healthy behavior—and remember that in this country, the cure for anxiety is (drum roll, please) . . . *more food!*

So try a more positive strategy! Compliment your child on good decisions, and empathize during the difficult times when her decisions are not the best. Whatever you do, remain sensitive to your child's need for affirmation and unconditional love.

Mealtime Chatter

When your child gives a lengthy explanation of how he designed a dinosaur from Legos, hang on every word. When your daughter gives a mind-numbing reenactment of a play that her friends wrote during recess, don't redirect her to her food. All too soon, you won't be able to drag more than "Uh-huh" or "Whatever" out of your kids! Mealtime chatter allows a natural distraction from the food so that the meal can progress more slowly and food satisfaction can more easily be recognized. Resist the temptation to tell your children to stop talking and eat. Why on earth do we do that? While most of us can relate, we may not realize how frequently we are sending mixed messages.

Chop Down Those Weeds!

One of our most important jobs as parents is to limit outside influences that threaten to strangle our child's ability to grow and thrive. Mealtimes are no exception! All electronic gadgets should be unplugged and turned off until the meal is over and dishes have been done. The TV and food are incompatible. The amount of time your child spends watching television and playing video games has a direct impact on his weight.

Every hour your child spends with his eyes glued to a screen is an hour that could have been enjoyed doing something active. While we address this topic in more detail in chapter 10, in the meantime, consider decreasing your family's television/electronic consumption. While your decisions may not make you a member of the "cool parent club," that's okay. The important thing is to raise a child who has a fit body and a healthy heart, as well as good habits that will last a lifetime! The rewards will be worth your effort.

Spirit Moment: Patience and Self-Control

As you teach your child to wait for hunger and to stop eating when sat-isfied, you are fostering the character traits of patience and self-control. Remember that children learn far more from what you do than from what you say. If they grow up with patient, self-controlled parents, it won't be much of a stretch for them to follow in your footsteps. Unfortunately, your child isn't too likely to learn such virtues outside your home. A current soft-drink television commercial loudly proclaim-ing, "I want it—and I want it now!" is typical of our society's attitude toward just about everything. Characteristics such as patience and self-control can't be purchased at Wal-Mart. They are traits that result from your relationship with God. Consider the words of Paul in his letter to the Galatians:

> But what happens when we live God's way? He brings gifts into our lives, much the same way that fruit appears in an orchard—things like affection for others, exuberance about life, serenity. We develop a willingness to stick with things, a sense of com-passion in the heart, and a conviction that a basic holiness per-meates things and people. We find ourselves involved in loyal commitments, not needing to force our way in life, able to mar-shal and direct our energies wisely (Gal. 5:22-23, *THE MESSAGE*).

Let's Review

What we've covered in the last two chapters represents the heartbeat of how to raise a fit kid in a fat world, so let's briefly review!

Portion sizes in our culture are out of control, and most of us tend to eat more than we need. It is essential that overweight children learn to eat less, but putting kids on a rigid diet isn't the answer. Instead of fol-lowing the trends of the culture, we want children to follow what their God-given body tells them about hunger and satisfaction. This model is best exemplified in young babies and naturally thin adults. As we progress on this journey, let's keep in mind that anyone can attain and maintain a normal size if they are willing to follow their God-given cues.

We introduced several concepts to help your child understand hunger and fullness. The Belly Meter illustrated an "empty," "satisfied" and "full" stomach, showing your child how to practice "0 to 5" eating. The Tummy Keys helped to walk you through mealtimes, with practical tips designed to help your child eat less food by paying attention to how her stomach feels. In Ages and Stages, we looked at practical tips based on your child's specific age and maturity level. As you put these tools and concepts into practice, your child will gradually eat less and will attain her natural, God-intended size.

As you consider what's been covered regarding hunger and fullness, we hope you are excited about a practical way to help your child slim down—without dieting! But perhaps you feel overwhelmed by all of this information or fear that you just don't have what it takes to help your child get healthy. Please don't give in to this deception! If you care enough about your child to read this book, then you have what it takes. Hang in there and continue to move forward. Before you know it, you will be naturally integrating these powerful changes in your family's life, which will impact your child forever.

As you read through our tips for conscious eating, you may recall times in the past when you have done the exact opposite of what we're recommending. There is a very simple explanation for any and every mistake you have ever made: *You are human!* For reasons we may never fully understand, God decided to choose fallible humans to raise precious children. Consider these wise words from Charles Swindoll:

> I can assure you that your failures will not doom your children to a horrible future. God's grace superabounds where sin abounds. Your love will cover a multitude of mistakes. This overwhelming responsibility is not so overwhelming when you recognize that *your children really belong to the Lord, and He will not fail you if you diligently and sincerely seek Him.*[6]

Don't dwell on past mistakes or fear the future. Accept that God hand-picked you as the parent for your child. He has uniquely gifted you for the task, and He is ready, willing and able to clean up after any and all mistakes as we seek after Him. So, as you continue to move forward, look up, and allow Him to direct each step.

Father, we thank You for our precious children. We feel so inadequate,
and yet we trust that You placed us here for a purpose.
Help our children to recognize the signs of hunger and fullness
that You designed. Fill us with Your grace so that we might be able to
make changes within our family without criticism or condemnation.
Lord, we seek Your wisdom to give us strength and to help our unbelief!
Amen.

May the Master take you by the hand and
lead you along the path of God's love
and Christ's endurance.

2 Thessalonians 3:5, *NCV*

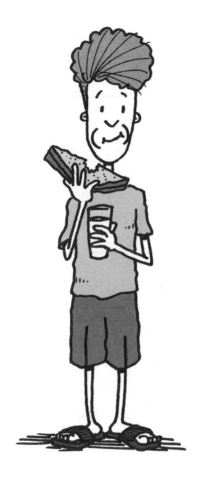

CHAPTER 5

GET SMART ABOUT FOOD FACTS

Practical Tips for Balanced Eating

Have you stopped to think about what really makes a food healthy? Is it what the manufacturers of packaged foods tell us on their colorful labels? Is a healthy food one that is low in fat, low in calories or low in carbohydrates? Is it food with lots of vitamins and minerals, or a lack of added preservatives? Are there really "good fats" and "bad fats"? And should you grill, toast, poach, fry—or microwave?

Trying to decide what's right for your family is enough to cause a headache! So we asked food connoisseurs of all ages, "What makes a food healthy?" Here are their replies:

- If it has Vitamin C in it, maybe, like apples. —*Gracie, age 6*

- If it tastes bad, then it's usually pretty healthy. —*Cody, age 8*

- A major thing that makes food healthy is not much sodium, grease or fat in the food. Veggies are healthy and they have none of those. —*Erin, age 11*

- If it says, "You can't eat just one" on the package, then it isn't healthy! —*Meghan, age 26*

- Healthy food implies a wide variety of foods. Nutritional value; natural vs. processed; any "pure" fruit, vegetable, grain, meat or fish prepared in a healthy way at home—not fried, and not something covered with breading or salt or that comes out of a package. —*Clarissa, age 41*

- Low carb . . . lots of green. —*Steven, age 54*

What a diverse assortment of replies! Clearly, what makes a food truly healthy is a bit more complicated than any one of these answers implies. Each hints at certain important elements, but a simple guideline for making wise food choices is hard to find.

As we search for answers, a trip to the grocery store can be quite enlightening. At the center of most groceries stands a "bling-bling" aisle—the one containing all the brightly colored, attractive packages that our children are drawn to like flies to honey. Spilling from the shelves are potato chips, cheese puffs, cookies, crackers and snack cakes galore, each boasting the *best* flavor at the *lowest* price with the most convenience you've *ever* experienced! We find ourselves wondering, *How did we ever survive without this new zip-lock bag that protects our potato chips?* Or, *Crackers, cheese spread, deli meat and dessert all packaged in one nifty container . . . how simple and cool for school lunches!* Or, *What? Cookies with chocolate chunks instead of chips—awesome!* Amazingly, these same packages almost always feature a one-liner with a splashy design that alludes to some health benefit. "No Trans Fat!" or "Low Carb!" or "30 Percent Fewer Calories!" all tell us that we can enjoy corn chips and bonbons with all the taste and none of the consequences.

On the other hand, the fresh produce department, with its apples, oranges, grapes, broccoli, lettuce and tomatoes, can be downright boring by comparison. It almost seems that more nutritious foods are left to sell themselves, while all the advertising hype is devoted to foods that have nothing much to offer, nutritionally speaking. Marketing strategies designed to compel shoppers to select items from the produce department are minimal at best.

With the entire marketing and advertisement world working against us, it's essential that we develop a practical understanding about the plethora of foods available in our fast-paced, microwave world. What makes food healthy *matters!* Instinctively we all acknowledge this, but the overwhelming food choices facing us make it seem easier at times to just forget about trying to figure out food labels—and order a Whopper and fries.

This dilemma is illustrated by Julie, an intelligent and independent professional with two children. "I am completely confused about food!" she exclaims. "One day I read that fat is bad. Then the next day I'm told that carbs are bad. Which is it?" Most of us can relate to Julie's confusion.

Don't give up! The process of making wise food choices for you and your child can be both enjoyable and easy to implement. The most important task is to develop a basic understanding of what makes food nutritious.

By becoming educated about what makes food healthy, we remove the sense of hesitation that leads to inconsistency. Lack of knowledge and foresight no longer cause us to be overly permissive with our kids, or to become overly restrictive and critical. Neither one is the desired goal.

Whether you need some basic education or a gentle kick in the pants to live according to what you already know is best, we want to offer some worthwhile guidance. The best changes are both subtle and slight—ones that your family will stick with in the long run. Again, when it comes to food, your children will typically imitate what they see, so rise to the occasion and set a good example.

Joanne began her journey toward healthy eating by incorporating gradual changes to her family's eating habits. "I started off by introducing some flashy new plates that were smaller than our old ones. The kids immediately noticed how colorful they were, but didn't even comment on the smaller size. It didn't take long before we were eating less without making it a big deal!"

She went on to explain that she applied this same approach to making more nutritious foods available for her children. "I knew we had to make a transition from fast food to more frequent home cooking. So my first step was to prepare fried chicken tenders and french fries—sort of giving them the 'fast food experience' at home, knowing that my version was lower in fat and salt. Later I made the transition to grilled chicken fingers and seasoned baked-potato wedges, two favorites that are now regularly enjoyed by our entire family."

Slowly guiding your child toward new food choices that offer a variety of flavors and nutrients is important. Food provides the needed fuel for our bodies to function correctly, and proper choices have an enormous impact on our overall health and vigor. Yet as your child learns to follow her God-given cues of hunger and satisfaction, it is also important to allow her to eat some of her favorite foods.

As we explore some food facts, we stand firm on the promise we made in the first pages of this book: We will *not* ask you to put your child on a diet, count calories, or develop a spreadsheet to keep track of how many servings of fruits, vegetables and grains your child eats on any given day. While every method of calculating food and nutrient intake may have some merit, the truth is, most of us don't have the time or energy to pull it off. It isn't that such tools are inherently evil, but rather that, on the grand list of parenting tasks, other things are a higher priority, such as remembering to give the kids a bath, making sure they have clean underwear, and helping them with their homework—not to mention loving them unconditionally! Plus, any time we start focusing on dieting rules or become obsessed with outward appearance, we may lose sight of the blessing of our precious, wonder-filled child.

Does this mean that we should give up on nutrition altogether? We don't think so. And since you're reading this book, we don't believe you think so either! So let's begin with a basic foundation of general nutrition and health. Then we'll introduce simple and effective ways to *adapt them so that they fit into your busy family lifestyle.* In the process, you can ease that vague sense of guilt over past choices as you see your child starting to eat and enjoy more nutritious foods.

What Makes Food Healthy?

The definition of what makes food healthy is often an elusive one, and the truth regarding nutritious foods might surprise you. The word "healthy" as defined by *Webster's Dictionary* is "enjoying health and vigor of body, mind or spirit" and "implies full strength and vigor as well as freedom from signs of disease."[1] With this definition in mind, consider the way some foods are advertised.

Breakfast cereal boxes grab the attention of our kids and state boldly on the front that they are "fortified with essential vitamins and minerals." These colorful treasure troves assure parents that the product is "part of a nutritious breakfast." Good nutrition? Many breakfast cereals simply provide vitamin-fortified sugar. The milk poured over the top provides the main nutritional value!

Another favorite of many kids (and their busy moms and dads) is a prepackaged meal consisting of meat, cheese, crackers, juice and dessert. The front of the package declares: "Excellent Source of Calcium," while a side label says the package contains a "100 Percent Fruit Juice Beverage" and an "Excellent Source of Protein." A more careful look at the small print, however, indicates there is a lot more to this dining dynamo than what is featured in the snazzy slogans.

Do these foods provide any real nutrients—do they give our kids "full strength and vigor with protection from disease"? Not usually. If advertisers wanted to be really honest, the packages would simply state, "Saves Time!" or "Tastes Great!"—and leave it at that.

On the other hand, consider foods your child might call "yucky" but which contain many great nutrients. Does that food meet the definition of "healthy"? Yes, but it's questionable whether a child can enjoy vigor of the body and mind when the taste makes him gag!

In Fit Kid terminology, foods that are good for us and help our bodies work better are called "beneficial foods," or wise food choices. We have quickly learned that there are no perfect foods that can do it all. So, when considering wise food choices, it is important to get the *right stuff* in the *right amounts*. Therefore, we are faced with the challenge of evaluating and choosing from a variety of foods to strike the balance that our bodies need. While it isn't necessary to "balance" every meal, we should try to create balance over the course of any given week's menu. With proper overall nutrition, our bodies function as they should, repair and heal injuries, resist infection, and avoid deficiencies that could lead to disorders and diseases.

Unfortunately, clever packaging and tempting conveniences often distract us from the truth about a particular product. Many advertisements highlight one supposed health benefit, and we often fall right into the trap. To illustrate, consider an extreme example: If you want your child to be on a low-fat diet and fat was the *only* consideration, then he could conceivably eat lollipops all day long . . . and think you were the greatest parent on earth! However, some problems would quickly arise. Lollipops are indeed low in fat, but they are also low in everything else—except sugar. Because he wouldn't receive essential nutrients, his growth would be impaired. He would have difficulty resisting infections as well as maintaining and repairing important body systems that he needs to function properly. He would also be subject to tooth decay, anemia and a host of conditions caused by vitamin deficiencies. It's probably obvious by now that his "low-fat" diet definitely would *not* represent healthy eating. While we are unaware of any lollipop diets on the market, some popular "miracle diets" and junk food packaging claims make about as much sense.

Common Sense Corner

Incorporating wise food choices into your children's daily menu may seem like an insurmountable hurdle, ready to trip you up before you even get started. "Leafy green vegetables—are you kidding? My child only eats cheese toast, chicken bites and Oreos!" If this is your child, *you are not alone!* Kids will be kids, which is why we encourage you to make small but lasting changes in your family's food choices. Over time, these modifications will bring you and your family closer to your godly goal of health and vitality.

As we reflect on food choices, let's employ our common sense by considering other parenting areas that require wisdom. As you make decisions regarding clothing and toy choices, you most likely consider the quality of the product as well as its appeal to your child. If you buy your 13-year-old daughter a pair of clumpy shoes that, in her opinion, look like "granny shoes," then she's unlikely to care that they are sturdy enough to last a lifetime! Parents are frequently called to perform a delicate balancing act between what our children *need* and what they *like*. Teaching them wise food choices is no different.

Yes, your child may refuse to eat some foods that are very nutritious and insist on something (like cotton candy) that is closer to entertainment than nutrition. That's okay! Aren't her clothing preferences a little wacky sometimes, too? However, with a little creative effort and knowledge, your child may be surprised when she discovers that (*gasp!*) what she likes is actually nutritious! Don't try to design the *perfect* diet. Going down that path will result in more frustration and guilt than success and satisfaction. Instead, based on the tips you find in the following pages, focus on simple, subtle changes that can be plugged into your family's lifestyle.

The Building Blocks

Food is composed of important nutrients—protein, fat, carbohydrates, vitamins and minerals—that are broken down through digestion and used to fuel and nourish our bodies. Some foods have only a few nutrients; others have many. As we said before, there is no perfect food that contains all the nutrients your child needs (and, if there were, he probably wouldn't eat it anyway!). The key to good nutrition is eating a variety of foods that, when combined together, contain all of the essential nutrients. In infancy this is fairly simple, because human milk and infant formulas offer a nearly complete diet. Once your child moves past infancy, however, providing the right foods in the right amounts is more challenging. In fact, depending on the age of your child, becoming a rocket scientist may seem simpler than feeding him a balanced diet!

As we explore nutritional information, remember that humankind has survived a very long time without food charts, serving-size suggestions or calorie calculations. God has blessed us with the innate ability to seek out the type and amount of foods we need. At the same time, if your child's regular choices are between a cheeseburger or fried chicken tenders, deep fried onion rings or potato chips, her natural taste for nutritious foods has probably become somewhat dulled. Let's awaken those innate sensitivities and broaden her food horizon, while teaching her to pay attention to her God-given instincts of hunger and fullness.

Powerful Protein

Daniel, a strapping 14-year-old, was asked what makes food healthy. His one word answer: "Protein." While he didn't have the entire picture, protein *is* required for growth, and it is essential for building and repairing muscles, skin, bones and other tissues. Protein also plays an important role in fighting infection and is especially important when your child is in the middle of a growth spurt. While considerable controversy exists regarding the optimal amounts of carbohydrates and fat in our diet, everyone agrees that an adequate amount of protein is necessary.

Where Is Protein Found?
Chicken
Dairy products (milk, eggs, yogurt, cheese, butter)
Fish

Legumes (dried beans)

Meat

Nuts and nut butters* (e.g., peanut butter)

Tofu

The Benefit of Balance

Without adequate protein, a child's growth, learning, development and resistance to disease are all impaired. An excess of protein, however, is converted to fat and may be stored as an energy source on the hips or abdominal area. Foods that are high in protein are often high in fat, so excessive intake can lead to weight gain.

Subtle Shift Suggestions

- Offer leaner meats, focusing on non-fried alternatives.
- Gradually replace fried chicken tenders with grilled or baked chicken fingers.
- For children over two years of age, make a gradual shift from whole milk to low-fat milk.
- Add nuts to cereal, yogurt or salads for extra crunch and extra protein.

Creative Carbohydrates

Periodically through the years, carbohydrates have been vilified, and there is no question that Americans, and our children, consume far too much sugar. Yet carbohydrates are an important part of our diet and provide us with the fuel that our bodies need.

Carbohydrates come in two forms. "Simple" carbohydrates are those sugars that are rapidly absorbed and provide quick energy, while "complex" carbohydrates take longer to digest, resulting in longer-lasting

---

* Peanut and tree-nut allergies are a common and severe source of food allergies. For this reason, they are not recommended for any children under the age of two to three years. In addition, if a family history of nut allergies is present, speak with your physician to determine if and when nuts may be safely introduced.

energy and more stable blood-sugar levels (as compared to simple carbohydrates).

Where Are "Simple" Carbohydrates Found?
Candy
Chips
Foods made from refined white flour (bread, crackers, muffins)
Fruit juices
Maple syrup
Sweetened colas/sodas
Table sugar
White rice

Where Are "Complex" Carbohydrates Found?
Brown rice
Dried beans
Fruits and vegetables
Whole-grain breads, cereal and pasta

The Benefit of Balance
Complex carbohydrates are full of vitamins, minerals, protein and fiber, providing appropriate energy and growth for children. However, excess consumption of carbohydrates (particularly simple sugars) can lead to obesity, insulin resistance and Type 2 diabetes.

Subtle Shift Suggestions
- Mix small amounts of whole grain cereal with your child's breakfast cereal, gradually adding more whole grain over time.
- Make silly-face sandwiches on whole-grain bread.
- Mix whole-grain pasta or brown rice with the original "all-white" versions, beginning with small amounts and then gradually increasing the amount of whole grain.
- Gradually decrease the availability of simple sugars such as candy, bakery goods and sweetened soft drinks.
- Instead of offering sugary snacks (such as candy or lollipops) as a reward, offer small toys such as those purchased at a dollar store.

Figuring Out Fat

Fat is an important energy source and provides insulation and warmth to the body. Fat provides antioxidants; carries the fat-soluble vitamins (A, D, E and K); and provides a great feeling of fullness and satisfaction because it takes longer to digest. In addition, fat contains fatty acids, which are used by the body for brain development, the formation of some hormones and the maintenance of good eyesight.

Let's dispel the myth that "Fats are bad!" We all need fat. However, all fats are *not* created equal. Fatty acids present in saturated fats are used in the production of bad (LDL) cholesterol, and saturated fats and trans fats can increase the risk of certain diseases, including heart disease and strokes.

On the other hand, monounsaturated and polyunsaturated fats may *lower* the risk of heart disease, high blood pressure, diabetes, digestive disorders and cancer. The key in making successful, healthy changes is to substitute the beneficial fats for the harmful ones.

The Benefit of Balance
Eating insufficient amounts of fat, as advocated by certain diet programs, can have an adverse effect on energy, growth, vision and learning. On the other hand, fat consumed in excess amounts can lead to weight gain, high cholesterol, liver and kidney disease, heart disease, and certain types of cancer. Per unit of weight, fat contains twice as many calories as protein or carbohydrates—which means it can easily contribute to weight gain.

Where Are Beneficial Fats Found?
Monounsaturated Fats
Avocado
Canola, peanut and olive oil
Cashews, almonds and peanuts
Nut butters (e.g., peanut butter)
Olives
Real mayonnaise

Polyunsaturated Fats
Most fish
Soy, safflower, corn and cottonseed oils

Where Are Less Beneficial Fats Found?
Saturated Fats (found mainly in animal products)
Butter
Cheese
Chocolate
Coconut
Coconut milk and coconut oil
Egg yolks
Ice cream
Red meat
Whole milk

Trans Fats (liquid vegetable oils that have been chemically processed to
    become solid at room temperature)
Many commercially baked goods (cookies, crackers, pastries)
Many commercially fried foods (French fries)
Many packaged snacks (butter flavored microwave popcorn)
Margarine products
Partially hydrogenated vegetable oil
Vegetable shortening

Subtle Shift Suggestions
· Begin using less salad dressing or select dressings with fewer saturated fats (but that still taste good!).
· Offer fruit, nuts, seeds or fresh vegetables in place of high-fat choices such as chips, cookies or pastries.
· For most cooking, use olive and canola oils instead of butter or
  other fats.
· Avoid deep-fried foods in restaurants that may be described as "fried
  in vegetable oil," as this often really means "hydrogenated vegetable
  oil," or trans fat.

Fast Food, Fast Fats

In our busy, fast-paced, "I need convenience *now*" lives, fast-food restaurants have landed on every corner. With very few exceptions, almost all of the choices on their menus contain substantial amounts of fats that are *not* in the beneficial category. A simple adjustment you can make is to reduce the number of times you eat at fast-food restaurants. It can be done—Kirstin and her family have a policy that limits them to just one fast-food outing per month. Now that may seem *radical*, yet making fast food an occasional alternative to eating at home will not only save you money, but it will also help you to reach your goal of having a trim, fit family.

Vibrant Vitamins

Vitamins play a crucial role in maintaining a healthy body. They help the body release energy from protein, fat and carbohydrates, and they play many specific roles within the body. The chart below gives us a sampling of some of the benefits attributed to various vitamins.

Vitamins	Benefits
A, B2	Helps maintain healthy eyesight
A, B2, B3, B6	Promotes healthy skin
C	Aids in healing and resisting infection
B6, B12, C, K, Folic Acid	Provides for blood production, clotting and increased immunity
A, B12, D	Promotes cellular growth

Pretty great stuff, those vitamins! Vitamins A, D, E and K are *fat soluble*, which means that they are absorbed and stored in fat. They are found in dairy products, foods containing fats and oils (such as fish and nuts), and in some fruits and vegetables. Vitamins B and C are *water soluble*. Vitamin B complexes are found in milk, meats, fruits, vegetables and grains. Vitamin C is found in vegetables and fruits.

Vitamin deficiencies can lead to a variety of disorders. For example, vitamin D deficiency can lead to poor bone development, while deficiency of vitamin B1 can lead to neurological disorders. Yet it is also possible to take too many vitamins. Keep in mind that vitamin toxicity is a risk, especially with children, so vitamin supplements should be used with caution—and only under the direction of your pediatrician or family physician.

Marvelous Minerals

Minerals are similar to vitamins in that they also serve many different and extremely important functions. A lack of—or an excess of—minerals can lead to a variety of diseases and disorders within the body.

Mineral	Benefits
Macrominerals	
Calcium Phosphorus	Build and maintain strong bones and teeth
Magnesium	Maintains muscle and nerve function, keeps heart rhythm steady, supports a healthy immune system, keeps bones strong, helps regulate blood sugar levels, promotes normal blood pressure, is involved in energy metabolism and protein synthesis
Chloride Potassium Sodium	Maintain body fluids and muscle metabolism; help regulate blood pressure

Mineral	Benefits
Microminerals	
Chromium	Enhances the role of insulin; plays a vital role in metabolism

Copper	Contributes to the development of bones and connective tissue
Fluoride	Helps prevent tooth decay
Iodine	Aids in thyroid hormone production
Iron	Necessary for the production of red blood cells and transport of oxygen
Manganese	Contributes to the development of bones and connective tissue
Selenium	Protects cells from breakdown
Zinc	Assists in healing of wounds; supports a healthy immune system

Below is a sampling of some foods that provide some of these marvelous minerals.

Food	**Contains These Minerals**
Milk	Calcium, Potassium, Iodine
Meats	Potassium, Magnesium, Phosphorus, Chromium, Zinc
Green leafy vegetables	Calcium, Magnesium, Potassium, Iron, Manganese
Fish or shellfish	Copper, Selenium, Iron, Phosphorus
Whole grains	Chromium, Manganese, Copper, Phosphorus

The appendix contains a complete listing of vitamins and minerals, together with the bodily functions they promote and their common food sources. A fun way to get children interested in more nutritious foods is to play games identifying the vitamins and minerals in different foods, and then explaining what these nutrients do inside our bodies. (In the Fit Kids Workbook at the back, several interactive puzzles and games will help your child learn which vitamins or minerals may help him see better, heal cuts faster or grow strong bones.)

Fabulous Fiber

Fiber is an un-digestible form of food that does not provide any calories or energy, yet it is essential to the health of the body. Sadly, fiber is often a missing ingredient in the American diet. "Insoluble" fiber passes through the body unchanged and is essential for proper functioning of the intestinal tract. "Soluble" fiber delays absorption of glucose, which improves blood sugar levels, and it also helps prevent cholesterol absorption. Appropriate fiber intake may lower the incidence of heart disease, high blood pressure, colon cancer, prostate cancer and obesity.[2]

Cynthia's 10-year-old son always complained of stomach pain. They had tried several over-the-counter medications and even a prescription medicine for acid reflux, all to no avail. However, once she increased the fiber and water consumption in his diet by adding in more fruits and vegetables, he had softer, more frequent bowel movements—and his stomach pain disappeared. Her son felt better "regularly" and so did she!

Where Is Fiber Found?
Brown rice
Fresh fruits (apples, blueberries and citrus)
Fresh vegetables (broccoli and green beans)
Legumes (beans, peas, lentils)
Nuts
Oats, barley
Whole-grain breads and cereals

Subtle Shift Suggestions
• Offer fresh fruits or veggies whenever your child is hungry. An added light touch of yogurt or ranch dressing may make these healthy treats more appealing.

- Take fruit or nuts with you when traveling in case you or your children get hungry.
- Sprinkle ground barley or oats onto salads, oatmeal, or even on a peanut butter and jelly sandwich for added "crunch"!
- Add ground flax seeds, nuts or wheat bran to cereal, oatmeal or yogurt.
- Eat the skin of fruits and vegetables when appropriate.
- Flavor water with fresh lemon or lime slices.

Wonder of Water

Water plays many important roles within the body and is essential for life. It is a part of every living cell and transports the nutrients found in food to each one of those cells. Water helps maintain body temperature, aids metabolism, helps get rid of waste and acts as a lubricant throughout the body. The body's supply of water must be constantly replenished—an adequate intake of approximately six to eight glasses of water a day helps promote proper digestion and metabolism. Lack of water, if prolonged or severe, leads to dehydration that may be life-threatening. Drinking too much water, on the other hand, can lead to an imbalance of bodily fluids.

Subtle Shift Suggestions
- Provide water at every meal until it eventually becomes the beverage of choice for your family.
- Carry individual-sized water bottles in a small ice chest in the car, and encourage the family to drink water more frequently.
- Help your child decorate a plastic, reusable water bottle to keep handy while playing outdoors.
- Consider making a "water only" rule for drinks in the car. This will encourage more water consumption and might eliminate some sticky messes!

Incredible Insulin

This little hormone has been happily doing its job for years, but only recently has it found its way into the limelight! Insulin is not a nutrient found in food; rather, it is a hormone produced by the body. Insulin has the incredibly important role of regulating the amount of glucose (sugar) in our bloodstream. A very low blood sugar level can cause seizures, brain damage and even death, whereas a high level can damage the eyes, kidneys and other bodily organs. So, insulin is essential for health!

After we eat, insulin is released in differing amounts depending on the composition of the meal. Insulin binds to cells throughout our body, allowing glucose to enter the cells for use as energy. When we eat sugar, our blood sugar rises, causing a release of insulin. The higher level of insulin then sends more sugar into the cells, the cells use it for energy, and our blood sugar level returns to normal.

The problem for many adults, and more and more children, is that this working relationship between insulin and glucose gradually breaks down, requiring increased amounts of insulin to handle the same amount of sugar. This imbalance is termed *insulin resistance* and is the first step down the slippery slope toward Type 2 diabetes. The cause of this is complex and not completely understood, but it is felt that several factors are involved: (1) a genetic component, (2) obesity, (3) a hormone (resistin) secreted by fat cells, and (4) lack of exercise.[3] Some of these factors, separately or in combination, interfere with the action of insulin. In the past, it was believed that weight gain was caused mainly by consumption of too much fat. However, we now know *all* calories (whether from carbohydrates, proteins or fats) consumed in excess of the body's requirements are stored as fat, which can lead to obesity, insulin resistance and diabetes.

To help your child avoid this dangerous cycle, it is important to provide foods that will not overtax the insulin-glucose relationship. Eating foods containing large amounts of sugar results in an immediate release of large quantities of insulin, while other foods cause a gradual release of smaller amounts of insulin. The effect of a food on the release of insulin is referred to as its "glycemic index" or "glycemic load." In general, the higher the glycemic index of a food, the worse it is for the body, since it causes more insulin to be released. Some examples of foods with a high glycemic index include most candy and simple sugars, white rice, baked potatoes, vanilla wafers, corn flakes and watermelon. Foods with a lower glycemic index translate into a slower release of less insulin; such foods include most fruits and vegetables, beans, lentils, oats, buckwheat, whole barley and peanuts. While we don't advocate regularly calculating these numbers for your child's intake, a basic understanding of glucose and insulin is an important aspect of determining wise food choices for your child.

Fortified Foods and Supplements

We also receive nutrients through fortified foods (such as iodized table salt, vitamin and iron-fortified cereals, calcium-fortified juices, fluoridated water) and by taking vitamins and minerals in pill form. While eating fortified foods and taking supplements can enhance health, it is better to consume nutrients in their natural form, as present in food.

The Food Pyramid

To help parents provide beneficial foods for their children, the Center for Nutrition Policy and Promotion—an organization of the U.S. Department of Agriculture—developed the food pyramid for adults and children, which is available at www.mypyramid.gov.[4] The food pyramid represents "science sense" and can be a helpful tool for learning more about nutrition, but we *don't* advocate turning eating into a legalistic exercise. If the food pyramid helps you to understand basic nutrition, feel free to utilize it. But please don't obsess over the number of servings of yellow vegetables your child is or isn't eating!

Medical Moment: The Deal with Diets

Diets, dieting books and dietary products are everywhere. Such diet-related merchandise ranges from the thoughtful to the ridiculous, lining the pockets of celebrities and charlatans, generating millions of dollars of income, filling the pages of popular magazines, and occupying an enormous amount of shelf space in bookstores.

Why do diet-related products create such a stir? How do they repeatedly entice us to spend our hard-earned money in the hope that—*this time!*—something might actually work? Well, most diets promise what we crave: structure and quick success. We want to be told what to eat; we want immediate success; we want a guarantee that it will work—and we want someone to blame if it doesn't! So, when a product boasts of these things with a money-back guarantee, we are tempted to throw common sense and money out the window.

While some diets have provided important health insights, even diets based on sound medical principles can have serious shortcomings. The problem rests in the impracticality of following these plans long-term in "real life." The same structure that we initially crave ("Just tell me what to eat!") may become irritating and inconvenient over time. Changes may bring initial success and weight loss, but then comes a trip to Disney World, an unexpected conflict or a party. Before long, counting calories or carbs may change from a welcome structure to an annoying set of legalistic rules. We tend to cheat a bit by "creative counting" or by convincing ourselves that the chicken salad sandwich at our favorite restaurant is *about* the same as the recipe in our low-carb cookbook. We may overeat "healthy" foods that are "allowed" or find ourselves alternating between binge eating and periods of "being good."

Rigid diet plans can adversely affect our children in many ways as well. The "rule followers" among us want to feel *justified* that we are doing the right thing. So if we put our family on a regimented diet, carefully purchase and prepare the right foods, and it still doesn't work, what happens? The temptation is to cast blame, either on a not-so-enthusiastic spouse, a well-intentioned grandparent or even our child. We can very easily and unintentionally convince a child that her self-worth is tied to her performance, weight or appearance. When that happens, the dieting—even if it results in weight loss—*is no longer healthy*.

Successful long-term changes, whether with finances, health issues or spiritual growth, do not come easily and almost never come from following legalistic restrictions. While such restrictions may bring quick success, the long-term consequences are often resentment, rebellion and weight gain. As we journey down the path of raising trim, fit kids, it is our hope that you will undertake simple, long-lasting changes that can be enjoyed and maintained by your entire family.

Putting It All Together

Whew! You've put a lot of energy into understanding the miraculous, intricate ways that our bodies work, and we hope you are feeling enlightened rather than confused! You need not become a registered dietician to help your child on the path toward making wise food choices. Instead, a basic understanding of nutrition will provide the information you need to make healthy choices when you are confronted with differing opinions, enticing advertisements or new "scientific" breakthroughs.

A large part of our journey has focused on eating the right amount of food based on the body's cues of hunger and satisfaction. The next step in raising children who are healthy and fit is helping them learn to eat "the right stuff." All of the nutrients provided in food—protein, fat, carbohydrates, vitamins, minerals and water—are necessary to help your child's body grow and function the way God intended. Paul does a great job of summing up what this healthy-eating principle is all about: " 'Everything is permissible for me'—but not everything is beneficial. 'Everything is permissible for me'—but I will not be mastered by anything" (1 Cor. 6:12, *NIV*).

As we reflect on the food facts discussed in this chapter, keep in mind that this represents only one aspect of our three senses: the *science* sense. There are dozens of excellent food and nutrition books on the market, but nutrition information alone simply isn't the solution. Understanding good nutrition is really the *easiest* part of becoming trim and fit.

The bigger challenge is finding realistic ways to incorporate beneficial food choices into our daily lives without causing full-blown family mutiny in the process! So, what *is* the solution? Do we give up and declare that providing nutritional foods for our children is just unrealistic? Definitely not! Instead, let's recognize that our "science sense" needs some assistance before good nutrition can become a reality in our busy, chaotic lives. As we also employ common sense and seek God's loving guidance, we will learn some simple, practical ways to close the gap between your child's current approach to eating and the one that you desire. In the next chapter, we will move from knowledge and theory into real life—warts and all!

Lord, thank You that You have made a broad variety of foods
that offer us everything we need to support our physical bodies.
Please give us the wisdom and insight
to consistently apply what we know is best.
Direct us in making small changes that will move us closer
to the healthy lives You desire for each and every one of us.
Thank You, Lord.
Amen.

It takes wisdom to have a good family
and it takes understanding to make it strong.
It takes knowledge to fill a home with
rare and beautiful treasures.

Proverbs 24:3-4, *NCV*

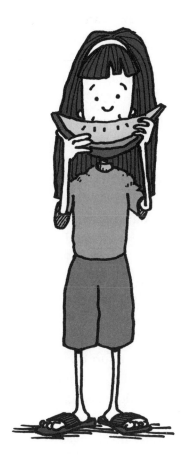

CHAPTER 6

SMARTS IN ACTION

Practical Tips for Making Wise Food Choices

As Saturday morning dawns and you roll over in bed to catch a few more winks before the weekend gets started, boisterous noise from the family room ricochets down the hall and destroys the last moments of sweet slumber. Sounds of teenage mutant Ninja turtles busting up bad guys on TV gives way to an authoritative voice telling the kids why they need to buy "Toastie Crunchies." You frown and wonder, *Why are the ads even louder than the shows? And why do they have to start so early?*

While some may dispute the value of Saturday morning TV, one thing that is *not* disputed is the connection between television viewing and its negative impact on our children. A whopping 97 percent of the food advertisements directed at our children on weekend mornings are for unhealthy choices—often a sugary breakfast cereal, a prepackaged "complete" meal-in-a-box or some sort of fast-food extravaganza that encourages kids to eat out.[1] How can roast chicken, steamed vegetables and fruit salad—fresh from Mom and Dad's kitchen—possibly compete with all that glitz, glitter and glucose?

They can, but not without effort on your part. You must continue on your journey using principles of *common* sense, *God's* sense and *science* sense rather than the world's *nonsense* of super-sizing everything! Instead of running out to get that new breakfast cereal, commit today to making gradual but profound changes when it comes to your family's eating habits. As you do, you'll rediscover hope and find the energy to pursue this exciting journey!

Preparation for Navigating the Waters

As God guides us in our quest to raise fit kids, He gives us a fresh vision—a grander view. Regarding all that we have experienced in the past, God says, "But forget all that—it is nothing compared to what I am going to do. For I am about to do a brand-new thing. See, I have already begun! Do you not see it? I will make a pathway through the wilderness for my people to come home. I will create rivers for them in the desert" (Isa. 43:18-19). What a wonderful promise!

God *is* doing a new thing—even now! Ruth related an eye-opening experience—one that led her to see the new thing God wanted to do in her family:

> I took my 14-year-old son, Steven, to a new dentist. As Dr. Harrison examined his teeth, she commented on the amount of softened or eroded enamel that made his teeth especially susceptible to decay. When she asked Steven if he drank much soda, I cringed, knowing full well the answer would be yes, and that the phosphoric acid in both diet and regular soda was the culprit. God had convicted me some time ago about the amount of soda being consumed by our family. This certainly was a wake-up call. I was finally ready to make some changes!

God used the situation regarding Steven's teeth to begin a new work in Ruth's home—that of letting go of a beverage to which she (and her family members) held a *deep* attachment. She didn't throw out soft drinks cold turkey, but she did share her concerns with the family and invited their input on what should be done. Steven suggested making a trade of sorts, substituting chocolate milk for some of the sodas. This turned out to be a good place to start.

Ruth reported, "The dentist actually liked this idea because Steven would get the vitamins and minerals that milk offers—even if it *does* have some added chocolate flavoring. At the same time, I realized I needed to drink more water in order to set a good example for my children."

As we discuss ways to incorporate healthy eating into your family's daily life, please accept them as recommendations—*not rules*. To assume that we could make a list of "do this" and "don't do that" rules that your child would obey like a trained puppy is unrealistic. We ask that you view our tools and activities through your lens of wisdom and experience with your own child. In the process, you will recognize some areas in which simple changes can have an enormous impact. Subtle shifts that can be continued over the long haul are far better than drastic changes that soon fall by the wayside.

Fit Kid Food Target

One reason why our attempts to eat healthy sometimes fail is that we get all pumped up for success and then focus *only* on what are commonly called the "good for you" foods. We try to convince ourselves that we really like celery sticks and hard-boiled eggs more than fried onion rings. But after a concerted effort, our dissatisfaction sets in and we find ourselves reverting to our former eating habits. However, this all-too-familiar cycle is about to bite the dust!

Today, as you seek to make beneficial choices for your family, you won't be hemmed in by preconceived notions and restrictive food lists. Instead, the changes you make will depend on your family's likes and dislikes. And your success will largely depend on your willingness to experiment and take some creative risks. Sounds like this could be fun!

The Fit Kids Food Target illustrates different categories of food, which will help clarify the difference between the more common, less healthy food choices and the more beneficial alternatives.

Taste-Bud Teasers

The first part of our target is an easy one to grasp—these are the "tasty" foods. Ask your 10-year-old why he likes his favorite food, and he's likely to respond, "Well, *duh!* Because it tastes good!" Unfortunately, many families in America have bought into the advertising concept that taste and convenience are what it is all about. Food choices based only on taste, with no thought given to *any* other benefit, are called Taste-Bud Teasers. These foods are nutritionally light, which means they have few if any of the nutrients or "building blocks" we discussed earlier. Unfortunately, in our fast-paced culture, many parents fall into the habit of offering Taste-Bud Teasers too much of the time.

Taste-Bud Teasers are usually prepackaged and are easy to open (like that bag of chips in your pantry). Their convenience taunts you into providing them for your kids, but they promise more than they can deliver because they contain lots of calories while providing little nutrition or long-term satisfaction. Advertisers capitalize on Taste-Bud Teasers by proclaiming, "You can't eat just one!" And the slogans

Figure 1
Taste-Bud Teasers

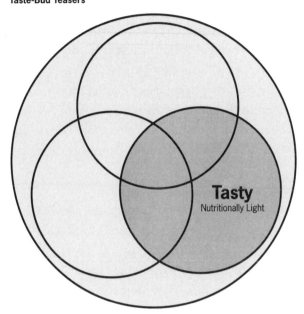

often work: Taste-Bud Teasers slip easily into your mouth when you are bored, watching TV, sitting at the computer, at the movies or in your car. But when you're *truly* hungry, Taste-Bud Teasers don't serve the purpose. You gravitate instead toward foods that are more gratifying and wholesome. Consequently, consumption of Taste-Bud Teasers can be a signal that your child is eating when he isn't truly hungry.

Record some of your child's Taste-Bud Teasers in the space below. Feel free to add some of your own.

_____

_____

_____

_____

_____

_____

_____

_____

In the Fit Kids approach, there are no forbidden foods, because we recognize that the very notion gives food an irresistible appeal. However, the foods we offer our children (and choose for ourselves) merit scrutiny if the goal is to be healthy and fit. It is harder to follow our hunger and satisfaction cues when eating Taste-Bud Teasers, because they provide little nutrition or physiological satisfaction. So while we won't say that your child should never have a Taste-Bud Teaser, we do encourage you to begin to examine these items more closely and evaluate the frequency with which you offer foods from this category.

Wholesome Foods

The next part of the Fit Kids Food Target is the area that is often the focus of traditional diets. These are the nutritious foods that many would consider to be "diet foods." In Fit Kids, we call these "Wholesome Foods." These foods are nutritionally dense, which means they have lots of nutrients, vitamins and minerals. They are benefecial food choices but often miss the mark in terms of taste and satisfaction. Some examples might include raw vegetables, skim milk, fat-free cheeses or dressings, or 100-percent whole-grain pasta. While these foods are filled with vitamins and nutrients and are clearly healthy, a sudden change to them may not provide the taste or satisfaction that your child is accustomed to.

Record some of your child's Wholesome Foods in the space below. Feel free to add some of your own.

_____

_____

_____

_____

_____

_____

_____

_____

_____

_____

Figure 2
Wholesome Foods

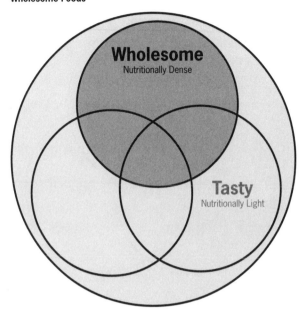

It's generally a mistake to load up the pantry with nothing *but* wholesome foods. You may have been tempted to do this in the past—you certainly aren't alone—and you may have also discovered that this change was met with a disgruntled attitude on the part of your kids, if not outright resentment. This well-intentioned, headstrong approach usually lasts only a short time and ends in frustration. But, fortunately, this *isn't* the end of the story. As we will learn, making gradual changes toward these choices may open the door to even *your* picky child enjoying more wholesome choices!

Gratifying Foods

In Fit Kids, we have a third category, called "Gratifying Foods." Sounds pretty good, wouldn't you say? Foods in this category are nutritionally fair, which means they are moderate in nutrients. They include "comfort" foods that typify the American "meat and potatoes" diet and make us feel as though we have had a real meal—we leave the

Figure 3
Gratifying Foods

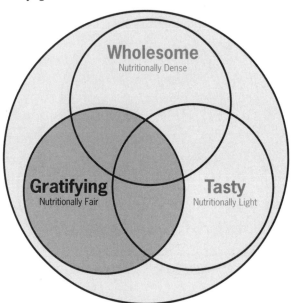

table with a sense of gratification. They are pleasurable foods, and in fact, many family meals fall into this category. But a nagging question often remains: *How nutritious was that meal?* When we honestly examine these gratifying foods with an eye toward health, we may recognize that their nutritional value is adequate but not optimum. Again, patience and creativity can save the day, as many of your favorite family meals can be tweaked to improve their nutrition.

If you feel you are offering nothing but Taste-Bud Teasers or doubt that Wholesome Foods will ever touch your child's lips, don't despair! Freedom *is* on the way! Our great God wants more for us than stewing over fat grams, carbohydrates and proteins—or deliberating over an "either/or" kind of menu. He has provided us with everything we need to delight our bodies and bring us vitality as well.

Whole-Body Pleasers
Now, let's look at the bull's-eye of the Fit Kids Food Target. This is the vital area that includes a wonderful assortment of foods that are big on

Figure 4
Whole-Body Pleasers

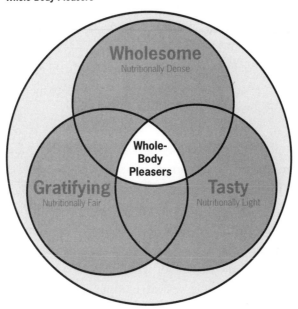

taste, big on satisfaction *and* big on nutrients! These are truly benefi-cial foods that we call "Whole-Body Pleasers."

Here, the tastiest, most wholesome and most gratifying foods over-lap in a wonderful category that offers the best food choices of all. As your child becomes willing to venture beyond the Taste-Bud Teasers, you are now ready to consider meals and recipes that not only taste good but also satisfy your child and help her body function well. These are "win-win" foods. Your child wins because she eats beneficial foods that she enjoys, and you win, because you know that the food you provide offers the nutrients she needs. The goal for you and your child is to dis-cover and incorporate as many Whole-Body Pleasers into your meals as possible. Here are some ways to recognize these Whole-Body Pleasers:

- They are foods you think about before you see or smell them— foods that you or your child truly enjoy when reaching that "0"!

- They are foods you appreciate from deep down, and they bring true physical satisfaction when you eat them.

• They may or may not be readily available—they might be something that you prepare at home, or a special dish at your favorite restaurant. Whole-Body Pleasers are *totally* satisfying foods you would go out of your way to enjoy. Unlike Taste-Bud Teasers, which provide convenience but little else, these foods are worth waiting for because they are properly prepared and can be thoroughly enjoyed.

• They are flavorful, satisfying *and* nutritious. Because of this, you might find that you are a bit pickier about what a Whole-Body Pleaser food is for you. For instance, instead of having just any old pizza with the works, your Whole-Body Pleaser might be a thin-crust, Thai pizza with plenty of chicken, onions and special sauce from that favorite pizza place across town! For you, it offers the benefit of wholesome foods *and* a wonderful taste sensation that leaves you completely satisfied and ready to go dancing!

Your child's Whole-Body Pleasers may evolve over time, and effort and experimentation may be required in order to identify them. They are "discovery foods." Be patient and ask God to help you and your child to discover some Whole-Body Pleasers together. Be adventurous and have fun in the process!

We have *lots* of food choices, with the average supermarket containing 40,000 items! Some foods are instant hits—a sudden burst of sugar isn't subtle—but others involve an acquired taste that may develop over time. Often, we assume that our children won't enjoy beneficial, healthy foods. But today we can begin to change that way of thinking. Consider Sheila's example:

We can talk ourselves blue in the face, but children will often imitate what we do. This was made crystal clear when I was teaching third grade. I frequently brought spinach salad for lunch and ate in the classroom so that I could catch up on my paperwork. The children had not tasted fresh spinach, so I offered them a leaf to try. At first they found it strange, "like eating tree leaves," but over time they kept coming back for more! For our end-of-the-year party, they voted to have my famous chocolate chip cookies and, you guessed it, spinach salad! All my students loved it and every year thereafter this "treat" was their special request. Occasionally a parent would call me and ask where I was getting those "leaves" their sons and daughters kept asking about.

With time and repeated opportunities for more nutritious choices, even *your* child may ask for spinach salad!

Children's likes and dislikes are usually learned behaviors. Japanese children are not born craving rice, fish and seaweed any more than American children are born with a taste for cheeseburgers. We influence what our children like to eat, even if we don't say it in words. As you discover new food choices, the Lord may surprise and delight both you and your child! God has plans for each of us and wants to lead us down a path where we enjoy a flavorful variety of nutritious foods. There are benefits He intends for us to receive from consuming the right stuff.

You may discover that some of your favorite recipes are Whole-Body Pleasers! Michaela and her mom evaluated some of their favorite meals for wholesome, tasty and satisfying qualities, and they discovered that their Mexican Extravaganza was a winner in each category. Bowls of grilled chicken, cheese, rice, refried beans (made without lard), lettuce, tomatoes, olives and onions were laid out buffet style, and everyone created his own burrito, nachos or taco salad. All of the choices were tasty, nutritious and immeasurably satisfying—and there were plenty of leftovers!

Each person's choice of Whole-Body Pleasers will be different, so no list can be used to determine "good" foods versus "bad" foods. If your child's favorite food has little nutritional value, then that fact alone will require some creativity on your part. Perhaps you could increase its value by including some healthy add-ons. Or you might consider offering it a little less often. This is a process that will evolve and change over time as her tastes mature and she tries new things. Encourage your child to evaluate food in a broader sense, appreciating food for the overall effect on her body, including her energy level.

List some of your child's Whole-Body Pleaser meals, recipes or foods. Don't worry about being "right" or "wrong" because you can add or subtract from this list as you and your child experiment!

_____

_____

_____

_____

_____

_____

_____

_____

_____

_____

_____

In the Fit Kids Workbook, we provide some fun activities to stimulate your child's interest and help him better understand the importance of Whole-Body Pleasers. Combining your child's hunger and satisfaction signals within the broad context of Whole-Body Pleasers is an important part of the road to health and fitness.

Total Rejects

Some foods are simply not worth eating because they contain too much of what we don't need and very little of what we do need. These are the too salty, too sweet, too fatty, too artificially flavored, unimaginative, don't-even-taste-good, yucky foods with no redeeming qualities. These are Total Rejects that aren't worth eating, aren't worth buying, and aren't worth having around.

Other foods fall into this category because they have adverse effects on your body. Are there foods *you* like but that don't seem to *like you*? For some people, coffee or highly spiced foods cause an upset stomach.

Dairy products may cause bloating or diarrhea because of lactose intolerance. People with celiac disease can't tolerate the gluten in wheat, oats, rye and barley. Chocolate can cause headaches or symptoms similar to a hangover. If your child has physical discomfort in response to a particular food, it may fall into the Total Reject category.

Another set of Total Rejects would include foods contraindicated (that is, not recommended) due to a medical problem. In metabolic disorders such as Phenylketonuria (PKU), certain foods are dangerous and must be avoided. Some children have food allergies, requiring that specific foods be reduced or completely eliminated. Speak with your child's doctor to determine whether a certain food must be avoided completely, or simply limited in amount. Peanut allergies are common and can be quite severe, so children under two to three years of age shouldn't eat peanuts or peanut butter. If there is a family history of peanut allergy, you should wait even longer to introduce them, depending on discussions with your doctor.

Other foods are Total Rejects because of age-related limitations. Infants and toddlers should not eat hard chunks of food, such as raw vegetables, fruit chunks (like apples), nuts, whole grapes or hot dogs because they pose a choking risk. Even when teeth develop, young children do not chew effectively, so food should be mushy rather than hard. A child's trachea (the breathing tube) is about the size of *her* pinkie (not *your* pinkie). Any hard, chunky pieces of food that size or larger can cause obstruction of the airway and even death, so they should be considered Total Rejects until your child is past the age of choking risk.

Ask your child what he considers Total Rejects, and list them in the space below, adding to the list anything to which your child is allergic or that causes an adverse reaction.

_____

_____

_____

_____

_____

_____

_____

_____

_____

Have Patience and Be Creative!

The lists that you develop will evolve and change as you continue this journey. Tina, a mother of three little ones, saw her own preferences shifting.

> My favorite Saturday morning breakfast—a Bavarian cream doughnut—became less appealing to me as I considered more nutritious options. Now, except for an occasional doughnut, I truly enjoy a breakfast with granola, almonds, steel cut oats and milk. The nutty, crunchy taste is _so_ yummy and oh-so-satisfying! My kids have willingly followed along, with my youngest child often enjoying a glass of milk, a fresh orange picked right off our tree, and wonderful whole-grain bread spread with peanut butter and topped with sunflower seeds and granola for extra crunch. We're all good to go for several hours, without the "sugar crash" that we used to experience after eating doughnuts for breakfast.

As the family's Whole-Body Pleaser list expanded, foods they once enjoyed paled in comparison to the new flavors God had led them to try.

Balancing Act
Regardless of what your child eats, encourage her to pay attention to her God-given signals of hunger and fullness, especially when she is eating something not all that nutritious. If she is able to stop eating when satisfied, she can occasionally enjoy those Taste-Bud Teasers with no harm done.

Ages and Stages
The age and maturity level of your child will determine how and when to introduce new potential Whole-Body Pleasers. Infants and young

children have little input regarding what they eat, so your main job is to provide—and model—beneficial choices. As your child matures, his food options will increase. If food with limited nutritional value is dominating his meals, cut down on the frequency you offer it and encourage him to develop other tastes. Older children will respond better to discussion, activities and explanations. The Whole-Body Pleasers concept will help children understand the overall benefit of foods and why some foods may be less available in the future. Evaluate your child's response as you introduce new foods. Rebellion and resentment might indicate a need to back off a bit, or that you might need a heart-to-heart talk to explore underlying issues.

Dining Out

Eating out can be a challenge. Large portions that emphasize flavor—to the detriment of nutrition—make dining out a tricky endeavor. If restaurant eating has been an important part of your family life, you may consider less frequent outings. Another obvious option is to choose more nutritious alternatives. Select restaurants that provide healthier options and serve some Whole-Body Pleasers. Be mindful that restaurant food may contain "hidden" calories in the form of fat, additives and too much salt. Educate yourself about content and methods of preparation, consider splitting entrees, and ask for a take-out box at the *beginning* of the meal to avoid overeating.

Some families try their hand at preparing their restaurant favorites at home. Earl and his family found this to be a popular experiment! Before he decided that dietary changes might be in order, every Wednesday night Earl bought two large pepperoni take-out pizzas, which were consumed with gusto by Earl, his wife and their two teenaged boys. However, sopping up orange grease that oozed from the pizza prompted Earl to think about a healthier alternative. The next Wednesday night, he purchased two ready-made pizza crusts, a jar of pasta sauce, cheese, pepperoni and lean meat at the grocery store. It took five minutes to assemble the pizzas, as he substituted a small amount of lean meat for some of the pepperoni. His sons enjoyed helping prepare the "gourmet feast," and everyone agreed that it was a wiser, more satisfying food choice.

Fast-food restaurants entice us with a "get it now" convenience and an abundant supply of Taste-Bud Teasers. If the need for convenience is what sends you to the fast-food drive-thru, consider fresh salads, grilled chicken and other alternatives that many franchises now offer instead of the "double-double combo" choices that are high in saturated fats. Or you might consider the creative approach taken by Marcie's family:

> To give us added incentive and help us cut down on our fast-food consumption, we turned a large French fry box into a bank, and every time we skipped fast food and ate at home instead, we placed some of the money saved into the box. Our savings accumulated very quickly, and before long we were able to buy something fun for ourselves. And we thoroughly enjoyed our home-cooked Whole-Body Pleasers!

Method of Preparation

Sometimes a food can be changed into a Whole-Body Pleaser simply by adjusting the way it is prepared. Many of us have developed an appreciation for the taste of fat and sugar. It might take some patience and creativity, but it is possible to gradually reduce the amount of fat, sugar and salt in our meals, while enhancing the flavor with spices. It *can* be done! For instance, baking seasoned chicken in the oven instead of frying it will result in great taste and is much more beneficial. Gradually replacing white bread, rice and pasta with whole grains will result in flavorful foods containing less simple sugars. The key lies in making subtle shifts rather than drastic, "in your face" changes. In time we can retrain our bodies, our minds *and* our taste buds.

When making changes, it is important to receive input from the kids, who *can* appreciate flavor and are not easily fooled by substitutes. If a certain recipe is just *too good* to compromise, then leave it as-is and offer it less frequently. Involve the entire family in planning some meals that include more beneficial food choices. Consider how much control we adults have over what we eat, and how little control our children have. Allowing them some decision-making power can go a long way toward getting the whole family to enjoy more pleasant and, hopefully, more nutritious meals.

Experiment with different methods of preparation, as well as a variety of seasonings and toppings. If some cheese sauce helps your child enjoy broccoli, go for it! If a little ranch dressing is needed to get your child interested in raw carrots or celery, that's fine. If your child is willing to try some milk with added chocolate syrup, then squirt it in! Getting your child interested in something other than sweetened soft drinks and a bag of potato chips is a *great* achievement.

Anything you can do to increase the nutritional benefit of some of your family's favorite foods will be a plus. Make sandwiches with whole-grain instead of white bread, add granola to a favorite sweetened cereal, use brown rice instead of white, or add ground-up flax seed to some yummy yogurt. Be creative!

Make Cooking Together a Family Fun Time!
Sheila and her family set aside time to make what they call a "Super Sunday Salad." They make it on Sunday so that it will be ready and available throughout the week. The goal is to find the heartiest, most colorful ingredients that won't go limp sitting in the refrigerator. These are some of their choices:

- Broccoli (cooked just a little, or raw)
- Carrots
- Cauliflower
- Celery
- Green cabbage
- Olives
- Radishes
- Red cabbage
- Red onion to taste
- Red peppers (as well as yellow, orange, green peppers)
- Snap peas
- Snow peas

The older kids help chop the vegetables, while the younger ones combine and toss the ingredients, placing them in a big storage bowl in the refrigerator. When it is time to serve, Sheila lets the kids add even more goodies such as mushrooms, fresh spinach, parsley, cilantro, sunflower seeds, garbanzo beans, red beans, avocado, pumpkin seeds, and so on. She dresses the salad with Italian olive oil and balsamic vinegar, together with additional herbs and lemon pepper, for an explosion of taste and a Whole-Body Pleaser!

Maybe you're thinking that your family is just not that into salad. No problem! Find something else that the whole family enjoys eating, and then find a way to make preparing that meal an experience everyone can participate in. It may take a little time and effort to find a good fit for your family—but we guarantee that once you've discovered your own family fun time in the kitchen, you'll never look back!

What to Drink?

If your child doesn't like to drink water, creativity is called for! Water should be available at every meal. To encourage drinking it, you might try introducing a new artistic cup, adding sugar-free "mix-ins," serving the water with crushed ice, or purchasing bottled water. Most of us need to drink more water, so if your water-hating child begins to take a few extra sips, give her a pat on the back!

Milk and Dairy Products

Children need milk each day. If your child doesn't like milk, you might flavor it or add it to foods such as casseroles, cereals or oatmeal—and remember to look for other sources of calcium, such as yogurt and cheese. Whole milk is still recommended for children up to two years of age (although those recommendations may be changing in the future). Beyond age two, switch to 2 percent milk, and then consider a gradual change to lower-fat milk. You may also use powdered milk in casseroles, creamy pasta sauces, meatloaf, smoothies and when making hot cereal.

Medical Moment: A Drinking Problem

Beverage choices have changed dramatically in recent years. Children used to drink milk, water and orange juice, with soda and tea only served on special occasions. Today, fruit juices, carbonated beverages, sports drinks, energy drinks and gourmet coffees are the norm. Milk and water are consumed in low quantities, often only when nothing else is available. The health consequences of these changes have been catastrophic. Carbonated beverages, particularly sodas (even diet sodas), are now associated with increased bone fractures in teenagers[2] and in decreased bone mineral density in older women.[3] It is scary to realize that what our children are drinking now can affect their health when they are grandparents!

Setting aside the detrimental effects of too much soda, fruit juices (often assumed to be healthy choices) contain almost as much sugar as soft drinks. Some energy drinks contain enormous amounts of both sugar and caffeine. And as more and more of these beverages with no nutritional value are consumed, those that *do* provide health benefits are being neglected. Any creative way you can replace less beneficial drinks with milk or water will yield enormous health benefits.

Fresh Fruits and Veggies

Because they are rich sources of vitamins and minerals, fruits and vegetables are great choices for enhancing your family's Whole-Body Pleaser category. It may take time and repeated exposure, but it *is* possible to get your kids to eat fruits and vegetables. Most kids aren't getting nearly enough of these, but fortunately it is an area in which children often respond easily to positive changes. A good long-term goal might be to provide fruit at every meal and vegetables at all meals except breakfast, although sometimes even that can be done. One grandma relates her favorite breakfast: "I microwave some chopped frozen spinach, top it with shredded Jalapeño Monterey Jack cheese, sprinkle on a little seasoned rice vinegar, then top the whole thing with a poached egg and some salsa. It's definitely a Whole-Body Pleaser."

Fruits and veggies are always great choices, but the method of preparation can affect their nutritional value. It is possible to cook all the health benefits out of vegetables or peel away the vitamins as we remove the skin. Canned fruits and vegetables can be higher in sugar or sodium, while fried veggies will be higher in fat. However, these might be good transition offerings as you seek to expand your family's nutritious choices. So hang in there—and congratulate yourself on making positive changes every step of the way.

Clean Those Pipes!

Everyone's digestive system needs fiber, but if your child loves sweetened cereals, a sudden switch to All-Bran isn't likely to succeed. However, gradually adding some nuts or fruit to his favorite cereal will help you win the battle over the long haul. Another option is to grind up seeds that are high in fiber, such as flax seed, and sprinkle them over other foods or add them to salads. Suzanne said she added a little bit of ground flax seed to Cream of Wheat, which gave it a nutty flavor and texture. This is a real fiber booster! It's also wise to provide whole-grain breads that are higher in fiber than white bread, even though you might have to add some creative toppings to catch your child's interest.

Dealing with Taste-Bud Teasers

The demand for Taste-Bud Teasers can be a source of tension within the home. Rather than sparking rebellion by ridding your home of them all at once, try these helpful tips.

- Remind your child to sit down at the kitchen table, even if she plans to eat a Taste-Bud Teaser—no more grazing on the run.

- Make a Taste-Bud Teaser more nutritious by adding a topping, such as a piece of cheese or lean meat, which adds physical satisfaction. Many family-oriented websites list creative recipes for snacks that will appeal to children—but be sure to use your newfound knowledge as you look for Whole-Body Pleasers.

• Since Taste-Bud Teasers appeal to our senses, put them out of sight so that they will remain out of mind! (And don't forget to put them out of reach of the kids!)

• If your kids want a snack and are truly hungry, tell them they may eat a modest serving while sitting down, with all electronic gadgets turned off.

• Since many Taste-Bud Teasers are appealing due to easy access, make fresh fruits and vegetables readily available so that they can be eaten with little or no preparation.

Whole-*Family* Pleasers

Positive, healthy changes can be counter-productive if they create a battle between you and your child. So allow her to have some foods that she enjoys, but in moderation (remember eating "0 to 5"). You can gauge how frequently you'll serve her favorites based on how beneficial they are. And remember, make changes over time. Success should be measured not by the end result but by gradual progress and the great attitudes maintained along the way.

Another very important principle is that these changes will need to be embraced by the entire family. If your slender 12-year-old eats ice cream every day, your overweight 7-year-old will expect to as well. If naturally thin Dad loves Big Macs and fries, so will his overweight son. It is unreasonable to deny one child a favorite food if others in the family eat it regularly. So it is essential to secure the cooperation of the entire family, including those who *aren't* overweight. After all, eating in a healthy manner is important for *everyone* in the family, regardless of weight.

Spirit Moment: Wisdom

As parents, we often feel overwhelmed as we attempt to raise fit children. Rather than exuding wisdom, we often feel downright foolish! Modern culture is little help because it regularly bombards us with messages that range from absurd to dangerous. Those we look to for leadership and advice—physicians, pastors, political leaders and teachers—often struggle to be the role models of healthy living that we desire for our children. And what messages do we, as parents, send to our kids? While we speak of the values we want our children to embrace, it is all too easy for our actions to promote social status, outward appearances and the importance of "having it all."

Wisdom combines knowledge and experience with common sense and insight. It allows us to discern *what is right*. A walk through any bookstore will reveal shelves and shelves dedicated to parenting. Why? Because wisdom is something that we parents desperately want and need! While many parenting books are wonderful resources, the *best* book on parenting (and life in general) can be found in the Bible, in the book of Proverbs. If this book were ever fully appreciated and embraced, those of us writing about parenting would be out of business!

Listen to some of Solomon's principles for living:

> My child, listen to what I say and remember what I command you. Listen carefully to wisdom; set your mind on understanding. Cry out for wisdom, and beg for understanding. Search for it like silver, and hunt for it like hidden treasure. Then you will understand respect for the Lord, and you will find that you know God. Only the Lord gives wisdom; he gives knowledge and understanding. He stores up wisdom for those who are honest. Like a shield he protects the innocent. He makes sure that justice is done, and he protects those who are loyal to him. Then you will understand what is honest and fair and what is the good and right thing to do. Wisdom will come into your mind, and knowledge will be pleasing to you. Good sense will protect you; understanding will guard you (Prov. 2:1-11, *NCV*).

Parents and children are constantly confronted with worldly information, lifestyles and role models that influence our everyday choices. The decisions that we make as parents, as well as those we avoid, have a profound impact on our children. As we reflect on making choices that will improve the health and wholeness of our kids, may we rely first and foremost on true wisdom that comes from God.

Through recognizing and obeying hunger and satisfaction signals, your child can learn to eat *the right amounts* of food. And as your family becomes willing to develop a fresh perspective toward eating beneficial foods, your child will begin eating more of the *right types* of food. These two positive changes will work together to everyone's advantage and good health. If you are in a situation in which you cannot select the type of food being offered, then focus on hunger and satisfaction. If your child is in full rebellion, refusing to acknowledge his hunger and fullness signals, provide some Whole-Body Pleasers and just stand back! Any ground that you gain is of benefit. You may take three steps forward and two steps back—but that means you will be moving forward, which is great!

Father, we turn to You asking for Your wisdom
as we strive to raise fit children.
Grant us patience and discernment as we learn together
to choose beneficial and enjoyable foods.
Help us to join forces as a family and to make the commitment
toward health that our child desperately needs.
Thank You for what You are already doing in our lives.
Amen.

The LORD says, "Forget what happened before,
and do not think about the past.
Look at the new thing I am going to do.
It is already happening. Don't you see it?
I will make a road in the desert and rivers in the dry land."
ISAIAH 43:18-19, *NCV*

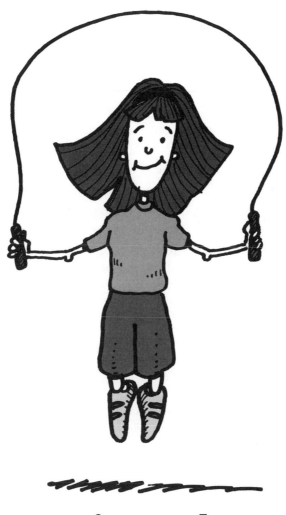

C H A P T E R 7

GET A MOVE ON

Increasing Your Child's Activity Level

Do you remember the carefree days of childhood? Summer vacations spent playing outside until dusk? Days were filled with games of Hide and Seek, Capture the Flag, and many more. We made forts, explored the creek bank, collected fireflies and ladybugs, played sandlot games—and, of course, got into a bit of mischief now and then! At the end of the day we often begged, "Just five more minutes, Mom! Please?" One thing we were as kids growing up—*active*.

Contrast this with today's techno-driven world, in which we are greeted by some pretty strange sights. Teenagers have wires protruding from their ears and bodies at seemingly every angle! Parents sit silently within five feet of one another, each with their own laptop computer. Two siblings share space on a sofa—one playing video games while the other's eyes are glued to her personal DVD player. If a space alien landed on our planet, it might wonder whether our species is able to walk and talk!

Mark, a discouraged dad, describes his experience: "When I come home from work, I look forward to some sort of welcome from my family. Instead, my son is sprawled on the couch, lost in music from his iPod; my daughter is playing a video game; the baby is mesmerized by the TV; and my wife is working on her laptop. Sometimes I feel like cutting off the power so that someone will notice I'm home!"

Over the past few decades, our idea of entertainment and fun has drastically changed. Fantasy sports now replace the real thing. Children of today can *talk* a good game, but they are far less likely to actually participate in one. Active ways of having fun have become nearly extinct. Many of our children have no idea what Kick the Can or Red Rover are, unless they are available on Nintendo Wii or PlayStation 3! Send the kids outside to play? With crime on the rise, many parents are fearful of encouraging the active outdoor play that we took for granted when we were growing up. The bright-eyed, rosy-cheeked excitement of children having fun outdoors has been replaced by the red-eyed, zoned-out look of those hooked on hour after hour of technology-driven entertainment.

Unfortunately, this phenomenon isn't limited to our kids. The techno rage has impacted our adult lifestyle as well. How many families go on a walk together after dinner? Can you recall when your house was totally quiet—no television, computer or other electronics—for an entire evening? A recent commercial depicts a father sending his children text messages, asking them to pass the salt at the dinner table! While a bit extreme, it does touch on a painful reality. With the explosion of technology, we have become more sedentary, more isolated and more overweight than ever before. We are in desperate need of a kick in the behind to get us all moving—so get ready!

Medical Moment: The Exercise Advantage

Consistent activity is *really* good for us! Regular exercise reduces the risk of heart disease, Type 2 diabetes, obesity, osteoporosis, breast cancer and colon cancer.[1] Physical activity also improves self-esteem and decreases anxiety and depression due to the release of endorphins, the "feel good" hormones from the brain that lift our spirits.[2] An added benefit of exercise is that it also takes us away from the television and the temptation to rummage around in the refrigerator.

Physical activity is beneficial because it increases metabolism—it revs up our engine! Without exercise and with too many calories, our bodies must figure out what to do with the "extra." As we discussed earlier, unneeded calories are stored as fat, and obesity often leads to Type 2 diabetes. Exercise, on the other hand, tips the scale back in our favor. Excess fat is burned for energy, insulin levels are improved, and glucose levels begin to normalize (even in those who suffer from Type 1 or Type 2 diabetes). Even more amazing is that this increase in metabolism continues to a lesser degree even after the physical activity itself has ended.

Regular exercise is indicated for all children and adults, barring any restrictions by your physician. The American Academy of Pediatrics (AAP) recommends that children engage in moderately intense physical activity 60 minutes per day. The AAP further recommends that the activities be provided through a variety of means, including unstructured play, chores, organized sports, recreation, planned activities and school-based exercise.[3]

Sadly, many of us aren't doing very well in this department. Recent studies have shown that our children are involved in more sedentary activities than ever before and are far less active.[4] A study in 2002 indicated that 60 percent of 9- to 13-year-old children did not participate in *organized* physical activity and 22 percent didn't participate in *any* physical activity.[5] To put it another way, over one-fifth of the kids were doing absolutely nothing!

It is obvious that some changes are necessary. While lifestyle changes are never easy, if undertaken with the right preparation and attitude, they can be fun *and* rewarding for your entire family. Beyond the health benefits, you can have fun together and build fantastic memories that will last a lifetime!

Let's Play!

This particular call of God on our lives is an invitation to *come play together*. It is clear what happens when our kids forget how (or never learn) to play—the kind of active play that involves climbing a tree or rolling down a grassy hill. While we don't expect you or your child to immediately rush outside and start doing Tarzan impersonations in the treetops, we do have a number of engaging ideas to get you going.

To parallel the AAP recommendations, we have divided activities into categories: unstructured play, organized activities and sports, school-based exercise, household chores, and planned exercise. An additional category, integrated activity, includes activities that can easily be incorporated into normal daily routines. As with introducing more beneficial food choices, the most successful approach will be slow and steady.

The best activity, like the best food, is a Whole-Body Pleaser—one that you and your child can delight in while maintaining a spirit of play. Keep in mind that for exercise to become a regular part of your child's life, it must be fun—which usually means you or one of his siblings will be exercising right alongside him. If you can find creative ways to make physical activity enjoyable, it will be one of the best changes you can make.

Integrated Activity

Some children are, literally, never still unless they are asleep. Others are so quiet that you must occasionally check to make sure they're still breathing! A simple way to break the "sitting on the bottom" cycle and help less-active children expend a little more energy involves activities that they won't consider exercise, such as the following:

- When your child is reading or doing homework, have her take a break for the "Seventh-Inning Stretch." You and she can then stand up, stretch as high as you can, shake your arms and legs— and maybe even sing, "Take Me Out to the Ballgame"!

- Take advantage of TV commercials for some "Moving Madness"! Jump up and down, wiggle around, do funky dance moves, reach for the ceiling, touch toes, leap-frog over each other—or do whatever your imagination can conjure up.

- Look for a *bad* parking space, as far away as possible from the store so that you have the opportunity to walk (or skip!) a greater distance. Even Jennifer's 12- and 14-year-old kids love it when Mom starts acting a bit "weird" as the three of them skip, hop or jump back to the car!

- Take the stairs instead of the elevator—and race to the top!

In the space below, list three ideas for increasing your child's integrated activity level:

_____

_____

_____

_____

_____

_____

_____

_____

_____

_____

_____

_____

Unstructured Play

You were a kid once, right? You may think you have forgotten how to play, but we bet you can learn again quite easily when given just the right encouragement. Mom, Dad, Grandma or Grandpa, this is your chance to shine and to be a kid again! Whenever possible, we want our children to increase their activity level through play. Exercise sounds hard. But "play" sounds fun! Playing *is* enjoyable and most kids love to do it. So get ready to take charge, be involved, and then watch out as the whole family rediscovers how to play again.

Outdoor Play

Games

The possibilities are endless depending on the age of your child, your climate and how much outdoor space you have available. Some standard but very fun choices include Frisbee, Hide and Seek, Hopscotch, basketball, soccer, jump rope, Red Rover, tag or having an Easter egg hunt (regardless of the time of year!). If you don't have a basketball hoop, use a garbage can or just enjoy dribbling contests. Don't worry about following the rules—just get active and have fun! Learn to play Frisbee Golf or create other fun variations on standard games. You can even make up your own games! Also find out which activities your child enjoys at school, and add his favorites to the list.

Seasonal Fun

When it snows, get everyone bundled up and head to the great outdoors! Go sledding, show the kids how to make snow angels, build a snowman, or have a snowball fight. If *you* participate, this will add a new dimension that increases the fun for everyone. Will you get wet? Sure. Will you get cold? Definitely. Will everyone have a whole lot of fun? Without a doubt! You will not only be creating awesome memories, but you'll be boosting your activity level and that of your child at the same time.

In the summer, head for the lake, a creek or the local swimming pool. Take a "Mommy and Me" class, have water fights, play pool tag or Marco Polo. Take turns retrieving objects thrown into the pool or have swimming contests. It is amazing the workout you can get in the water! If no pool is available, run through the sprinkler, or have an old-fashioned water fight in the backyard with squirt guns or the water hose. Remember, *anything* that has you and your child smiling and moving together is a winner!

A Grand Adventure

Most children love adventures, and hitting the trail for a day hike can be both fun and exciting. Perhaps you'll take a trek on an official hiking trail or have a simple adventure into the woods behind your house! Take a plastic bag or lightweight backpack to collect treasures on the way (if you are in a park or a nature preserve, be sure to follow any rules about not disturbing the natural habitat!). You might decide to bring a field guide of animal tracks to help you identify what night-time visitors have been in the area, or check out a book from the library to help you recognize the types of birds or trees that you might encounter on your adventure. To enhance your experience, bring a few creative items such as a compass, cargo jacket or a cheap fishing vest. And don't forget to pack those beneficial food choices, along with plenty of water. You and your kids are going to work up quite a thirst!

Younger children will enjoy participating as well. To avoid boredom, let each person take turns being the "leader"—or have everyone pretend to be walking on the moon, taking big, bouncy, slow motion steps to mimic the lack of gravity. Or add a game of Leapfrog as you go. Don't hesitate to get dirty; you can always wash up later!

A scavenger hunt is another great adventure your kids will enjoy. Make a list ahead of time of items that are sure to be found. Be creative—not all items need to be collectible. One of the clues on the hunt might be to "Use all your senses to find the sound of a bird, the feel of a caterpillar, the smell of a flower." Another variation is to incorporate some activities into the hunt, such as having a "finish line" to sprint toward after all the items have been found. Healthy competition is sure to build some lasting memories!

A truly grand adventure is called "Geocaching," which has become a big hit among many adults and kids who enjoy using techie toys and being outside at the same time. Using a GPS (Global Positioning System) and coordinates downloaded off the Internet, you can embark on a quest for a "treasure" left by another treasure hunter. You sign onto the website, enter your zip code and then go searching! The rule is, once you locate your treasure, you must then leave something behind for the next treasure hunter—CDs, books, toys or anything else you deem a treasure. Many spots even have a "guest book" to sign once you've unearthed your treasure! There are literally thousands of treasures "hidden" within any city, just waiting for you and your child. To find out more, visit http://www.geocaching.com.

Go for a Spin

You never forget how to ride a bike, right? Well, now is the time to prove it! Cycling provides great cardiovascular conditioning, while helping you steer clear of most orthopedic problems associated with jogging and running. So if your neighborhood isn't appropriate for bicycling, then scout for some nearby flat areas with little traffic (many cities have bike trails you can check out). Adding some desirable accessories to your child's bike can make it fun: a water bottle, basket, handlebar decorations or a playing card to click against the spokes. An odometer can make your ride more exciting as you challenge yourselves to ride a little farther with each outing.

Interactive Toys

Look for outdoor toys that involve movement, such as tricycles, bicycles, toy push lawnmowers, pogo sticks, roller blades, or a bat and ball. Let children help to make their own toys. Homemade "kites" fashioned from plastic grocery bags can be flown even without a breeze! Or make your own "bowling alley" using plastic drink bottles and a kickball. Check the library or the Internet for more ideas about inexpensive, homemade family-fun activities.

Playgrounds and Parks

Kids love a good playground! During the week, visit the park nearest your house. Then consider a longer drive to your favorite park on weekends and include a picnic. Play Hide and Seek or tag, fly a kite, or throw the Frisbee! Use your imagination to create a make-believe land of pirates, princesses, spaceships, fairies or dinosaurs. Instead of taking along a book to read, follow your child down the slide. Whatever you do, have a great time together!

Skates, Skateboards and Rollerblading

Most teens and preteens love catching the action at a local skateboard park or skating rink. Many skating facilities have activities for different ages on certain nights, so find a time that is appropriate for your child. If she approves, you could become her "sports photographer" and help her develop a photo album of her best action shots. Your child may not admit it, but she will be flattered by your interest! If skates and rollerblades can be used on the street, look for safe areas where your child can strut her stuff. And since safety is important, helmets are a must and, depending on the activity, other protective pads may be needed.

Local Parks and Recreation Department

Don't forget to check out your local Parks and Recreation Department. They usually sponsor all sorts of fun classes and activities, such as nature hikes, bird-watching tours, creek walks and even family bicycle outings.

In the space below, list five outdoor activities that you and your child can enjoy together:

_____

_____

_____

_____

_____

_____

_____

_____

_____

_____

Indoor Play

Obstacle Course

Collect all the pillows and sheets in your house, and build an indoor adventure! You can stretch sheets over furniture to form tunnels, pile pillows to jump over, and roll up blankets on the floor to be a "tightrope" to walk across. Add a "challenge task" at designated spots, such as performing 10 jumping jacks or doing a somersault at the end of the tunnel. Take turns designing the course, and time each other to see how long it takes each family member to get from start to finish. Your housecleaning may suffer a bit, but the laughs (and the exercise) will make up for it!

Outdoor Games Brought Inside

Many active games, such as Hide and Seek, jump rope and scavenger hunts, can be modified to make them suitable for playing indoors. If you have access to safety mats and enough space, indoor gymnastics (such as somersaults and cartwheels) can be lots of fun. Again, your child will enjoy it more if you are an active participant!

Dance and Movement Videos and DVDs

Activity videos of all kinds—for children and adults—are readily available and can be a great way to get moving on a rainy day. Many popular children's characters have their own dance or exercise videos, so let Elmo or Dora lead the way! Choose those that are more creative and fun, rather than work. Children are interested in having fun, *not* in "making it burn." If you have to use the TV to babysit your child while you prepare dinner, then consider having him watch an exercise video to assuage some of your guilt—and boost his activity level!

Dance, Dance, Dance!

Turn on some praise music or some of the "oldies" and start dancing! Seeing Mom or Dad "shaking their booties" might be a shock to the young folks, but they will surely join the festivities. A fun way to encourage dancing is through commercially available dance pads, which plug into your computer. All you have to do is follow the pattern on the dance pad to learn some great new moves! Dance pads featuring current Christian musicians are also available, as is a Veggie Tales version.

One active mom, who enjoys rainy day *Dance Praise* workouts with her children, said, "We get the best of both worlds: dancing, worshiping God, laughing together—all while using the computer! If you can't beat 'em, *join* 'em!"

Indoor Playgrounds

Play areas for kids are available all over the place—in shopping malls, fast-food restaurants, arcades and as stand-alone recreational facilities. Some play areas may not be safe for younger children at certain times (such as Saturday evenings), but they might be perfect on a weekday morning. Plan your food options ahead of time so that you and your child can make beneficial choices.

Bowling Alleys

Kids and adults of all ages can enjoy the bowling alley. Most have a bumper guard that can be raised to allow even very young kids to play without fearing the gutter ball. (Many adults might also benefit from a little bumper-guard assistance!) Bowling alleys typically sponsor youth leagues, so this might be an opportunity for her to shine if she loves bowling. Don't forget the camera!

In the space below, list five indoor activities that you and your child can enjoy together:

_____

_____

_____

_____

_____

_____

_____

_____

_____

Organized Activities and Sports

Organized activities and sports can be a great way for your child to have fun *and* be consistently active. But before you sign up for a group sport, take into account the expense involved, the convenience and time commitment factors, and your child's weight and any physical limitations he might have. An extremely overweight child may feel embarrassed about certain outfits (such as a dance leotard or swimsuit), and some overly competitive activities might be inappropriate for overweight kids. If you aren't certain, talk with your child's doctor.

If the time and/or expense involved seem like an insurmountable barrier, consider creative options. And consider how Morgan, Julie's mom, solved the money issue.

Our daughter Julie attended a birthday party at a karate center, and then starting begging us to enroll her in classes. We thought it was a great idea but just didn't see how we could pull it off. Our budget was really tight due to Jason's recent job transfer, and I felt strongly that I needed to remain at home rather than getting a job elsewhere. After we prayed about it for a few weeks, God showed us a wonderful solution—if we dined out three fewer times each month, the cost of our classes would be covered. Julie was able to increase her activity, we all ate better, and we actually had a little money left over!

We can all learn from Jason and Morgan's example. Seeking God's guidance for each and every concern is always wise.

Team Sports

Team sports help kids forge great friendships and learn the value of teamwork, and they promote fitness. Possibilities include soccer, basketball, softball, tennis, volleyball, baseball and swim teams (the Parks and Recreation Department usually offers a variety of options for specific age groups). Be sure to consider your child's ability level when choosing a particular sport or league.

Karate and Martial Arts

Karate schools, or *dojos*, are popular throughout the country. Children can develop skills in martial arts and self-defense and also gain confidence while benefiting from regular exercise. The individual instruction is particularly beneficial to kids with attention issues, and some centers even allow children and parents to train together.

Individualized Activities

Many communities offer a variety of opportunities for individualized activities, including gymnastics, dance theaters, golf, tennis, movement classes and swim lessons. The Parks and Recreation Department, local community centers and the YMCA often have lessons for children or adults, as well as times for "free play" that can be enjoyed by the entire family.

In the space below, brainstorm (with your child!) two or three organized sports or activities that he could be involved in. Choose one together, and go for it!

_____

_____

_____

_____

_____

_____

_____

_____

_____

_____

_____

School-Based Exercise

A generation ago kids attended PE class every day and enjoyed dodge ball or jump rope on the playground during daily recess. After 20 minutes of hard play, we were sweaty, panting and desperately wanting a drink of water! Unfortunately, those days are long gone for most of our kids. Physical education for many has been reduced to only one day per week, and even this minimal requirement often disappears by the middle-school years. Recess is often an optional privilege that may be taken away for incomplete class work. On rainy days, outdoor recess activities may be replaced by a movie or television. So what can we do?

- If your child loses recess privileges, ask the teacher how you can support her concerns about your child academically or behaviorally, and then ask for the teacher's support in providing your child the opportunity to be more active. Explain that you are concerned about his lack of exercise, and discuss whether other means of discipline might be feasible.

- Encourage your child to go outside for recess whenever she has the opportunity. Most teachers are more than willing to support this, knowing that the more active kids often do better academically *and* behaviorally.

- Consider choosing physical education as an "elective" for your child, if this is an option. Obviously, you'll need to think about your child's greatest needs, as well as the other electives available, before you make a decision.

- Get involved! Whenever possible, be active in your child's school so that you can have a voice in decisions involving physical education and exercise opportunities.

In the space below, list two to three things you can do to boost your child's activity level at school:

_____

_____

_____

_____

_____

_____

_____

_____

_____

_____

_____

_____

Household Chores

Performing chores is one way for your child to increase his activity level and be productive at the same time. While you probably aren't in a position to send your kids out to milk the cows, you can help get them moving by giving them household tasks to complete! Of course, which chores you delegate will depend on the age and ability level of your child.

Clean Up, Clean Up

Younger children often enjoy helping around the house. Make a game of it: Ask your child how quickly she can pick up 10 items and put each one in its proper place. Then give her a breather and you do it. Before you know it, the job will be done, and you both will have enjoyed the game and the benefit of physical activity.

Laundry

If your home is like some, you may have "Mt. Never Rest" right under your nose—it's the pile of laundry that never seems to end! Rally the troops, and tackle Mt. Never Rest together. Make it a game so that everyone can participate. "Everyone grab five things to fold—let's see who can be fast *and* neat!" "How quickly can you run these dirty things down to the laundry basket? I'll time you!" Younger children can help sort dirty laundry, middle-school kids can dump clothes into the washing machine or dryer, and teens can do the whole thing. Remember to give lots of praise both for the physical activity as well as for their willingness to participate.

Spring Cleaning

As a team, the challenge for the family is to accomplish their very own Mission Impossible: to make the walls, doors, window sills and trim *shine*! Each person is assigned a "zone"—a bedroom, bathroom, dining room or family room (of course, assign the youngest ones a smaller area). The goal is to make each zone spotless by cleaning the walls, doors and doorframes, windowsills, and baseboards. For younger children, provide cloths pre-dampened with furniture cleaner or window spray. Everyone wins when the entire house is sparkling! Again, reward the effort by doing something fun that all will enjoy.

Yard Work (and Play)

Working outside is a great way to be active and have fun. Having your kids sweep the walk, rake leaves (then jump in them), plant flowers or pick up clutter is a great way to encourage exercise. Why? Because they're active without even realizing it! Younger children can enjoy toy gardening and yard tools, while older kids can use the real thing. Take breaks for an impromptu game of soccer or croquet. When the entire family participates, outdoor "work" will seem more like play. Design an outdoor version of "Mission Impossible" or purchase neon-colored "jack-o-lantern" leaf bags to provide an extra dose of fun.

In the space below, list three household chore activities that your child can participate in.

_____

_____

_____

_____

_____

_____

_____

_____

_____

_____

_____

_____

_____

Planned Exercise

When we consider planned exercise, thoughts of aerobics or a stationary bicycle may pop into our minds. Rest assured—we *aren't* going there! If enough other areas of activity are utilized, then planned exercise should be only a small part of the entire picture. Still, it needs to be fun and enjoyable. Focus on exercise that promotes interest, *not* resentment, and that can be continued and enjoyed over the long haul.

Family Walks

Walking together is a great way to get fit and enjoy family fellowship at the same time. The key is creativity, because children (and adults) quickly become bored at walking "laps." Discover different places to walk, and then let the kids rank them in order of preference, highlighting different routes on a map and keeping track of all the trails you complete. But don't limit yourself to formal walks: When dining out, park several blocks from the restaurant so that everyone can stretch their legs before—and after—the meal. And on rainy days, indoor malls are great places to walk and talk together.

Exercise Equipment

While many adults loathe the stair-stepper, children often find exercise equipment fun. If that's the case with your kids, seize the opportunity! Try creative ways to spice things up: Take turns rotating from the treadmill to the stair-stepper, and then add a few jumping jacks. Make certain that your child is old enough to safely use the equipment, and provide appropriate supervision.

Walk the Dog

Have your child regularly participate in exercising—and playing with—the dog to make sure that both the dog *and* the child are active! And don't forget to have your child bathe and feed the dog, which will help him to learn about the responsibility of caring for pets.

Join a Gym!
If finances permit, joining a gym or the local YMCA can be enjoyable for the entire family. Many gyms feature special programs, racket sports, court games, all manner of exercise classes, workout equipment—even rock climbing!

In the space below, list five types of planned activity that you and your child can enjoy together.

_____

_____

_____

_____

_____

_____

_____

_____

_____

Common Sense Corner

Remain levelheaded as you consider ways to increase your child's activity. The exercise industry makes a fortune every January as everyone rushes out to purchase equipment and clothing to fulfill their latest New Year's resolution! And yet, the expensive treadmill often ends up as a place to hang the laundry, while the aerobics outfits get shoved to the back of the closet or donated to Goodwill. Rather than going overboard in your effort to become more active, make simple changes that can become a regular part of your family life (you really don't need matching outfits to ride bicycles together!).

At the same time, be creative. If you tell your child in a bored tone of voice, "We need to go for a walk and get some exercise," she isn't likely to be too excited. On the other hand, if you say, "Hey, let's pack a bag and go on an adventure!" she is likely to perk up and get interested in a hurry.

Children's magazines and the Internet offer many ideas for activities. As you fire up your creative juices, the possibilities for you and your child are endless!

Tools to Improve Activity

The hardest part of any new endeavor is the first step: moving from theory to action. It is easy to read about how to increase your child's activity and think to yourself, *These are some really good ideas!* The real challenge is to take action, so here are a couple of tools to help you get started.

The Fun Jar

Write activity choices on slips of paper and place these into the Fun Jar. You may have several jars for different categories (rainy days, outdoor recreation, and so on). Each day, have your child randomly choose one slip. Or you may "preview" the paper slips before your child chooses, allowing activities for which you have time and availability. After completing the activity, glue notes or a snapshot onto a special calendar or journal, stating what you did and how much fun it was. This is a wonderful way to record some shared memories *and* to track your physical activity!

Pedometer

Pedometers can be a fun and effective way to help kids get excited about stepping up their physical activity. Many schools utilize pedometers as a part of physical education, and the effect on kids is amazing! Many are reasonably priced and come in kid friendly colors. One word of caution, however: Remember to *keep it fun*. The number of steps your child takes should not be part of a rigid exercise program or cause for criticism. Simply use a pedometer as a way to interest your child in increased activity.

The Motion Monitor

Kids love achievable goals and frequent rewards. Simple tasks such as brushing their teeth are often met with a resigned, tired "Okay, fine"—until a brightly colored sticker becomes a reward. Suddenly, those eyes perk up and a spring enters his step: "Can I have a Spider Man sticker if I do a really good job?" In the same way, the Motion Monitor allows you to set achievable goals, provide those cherished rewards and chart your child's progress. Our example below lists favorite activities, with space to place a sticker each time the activity is completed. We have also listed a sample "wish list" for rewards. You will, of course, want to individualize your Motion Monitor to address your child's needs, interests and personality.

Your child's Motion Monitor might be a wipe-off chart, which can be found in the school supplies section of most stores, or just a sheet of paper. Ask your child which activities she wants to list and also include one or two surprises that might catch her interest. Next, decide on weekly goals as well as the value of the stickers and the prizes. Establish smaller prizes that can be attained fairly quickly as well as more expensive rewards that take more persistence to merit. Enlist your child's help in finding some fun, colorful stickers that will fit in the boxes. Finally, put it all together and find a prominent place where you can display your child's Motion Monitor.

Activity	Mon	Tue	Wed	Thu	Fri	Sat	Sun
Jump rope							
Hopscotch							
Sweeping the sidewalk							
Riding my bike							
Practicing karate							
Walking on treadmill							
Playing basketball							
Skipping							
Dancing							
Going for a walk							

My Goal for the Week:_____
I will receive _____ extra stickers if I meet my goal.
My wish list: *(Sample)*

1. Webkinz stuffed animal   = _____ stickers
2. Box of dominoes   = _____ stickers
3. A basketball   = _____ stickers
4. Softball glove   = _____ stickers
5. Magnetix kit   = _____ stickers
6. Gift card at my favorite store = _____ stickers
7. Bicycle horn   = _____ stickers

Spirit Moment: Joy

Making behavioral changes within a family can be a daunting challenge, and increasing a child's activity level is no exception. Before our children were born, we may have visualized a future with pillow fights, tickling and giggling, funny jokes and endless hours of meaningful memories. But after becoming parents, some of the fun may fade and raising children can become all work and no play. An important way to bring back the fun in your family is to ask God to show you the humor in each and every situation, and allow Him to reawaken your joy.

Jill recalls such an experience.

We were on our way out the door, grabbing backpacks and homework and school snacks . . . you know the picture. I turned to put the dog outside, and there, in the middle of the floor, was a big, huge puddle. I just wanted to *scream*! I knew I had to clean it up, which would make the kids late for school and me late for work. The whole day was starting off on the wrong foot! I shut my eyes and prayed, "Lord, please help me see the humor here." As I opened my eyes, something about Sherlock's long, droopy ears and big, sad eyes, knowing he was in *big* trouble, just made me laugh. The kids looked at me in surprise, then looked at the dog . . . and they started laughing, too. Sherlock sheepishly stayed in the corner, trying to figure out what was going on! When I finally got my sons to their classrooms and told their teachers the reason for their tardiness, we all had a good laugh. Even now, the memory of that poor dog's pitiful expression brings a giggle!

Through her simple prayer, Jill recognized the fun in a frustrating situation. The truth is, the twists and turns of our crazy lives would often be hilarious if viewed on a sitcom, but we don't find the craziness funny because of our perspective—when we are at the center of the storm, the humor is tougher to see. A wise person once said, "Blessed are they who can laugh at themselves, for they shall never cease to be amused." As you develop a plan for increased activity, remember to make it fun and learn to laugh together. In the process, your child will learn to roll with the punches and you will begin to experience more of the true joy of parenting.

FIT KIDS TRIANGLE

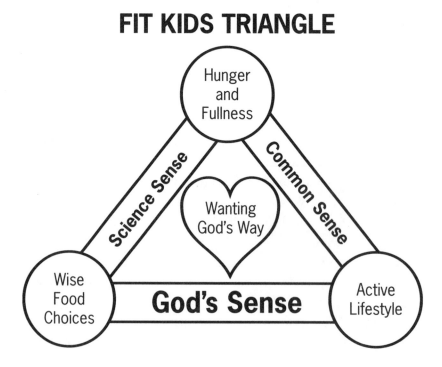

Give yourself a pat on the back as you review your progress using the Fit Kids Triangle as a guide. You've made it through the three different aspects of raising fit kids in a fat world: (1) helping your child eat the right amount of food through listening to the internal cues of hunger and satisfaction, (2) helping your child make wise food choices, and (3) helping your child increase her activity level. Binding these together are the three senses (*common* sense, *God's* sense and *science* sense) that allow you and your child to make informed, godly decisions. When faced with obstacles or when temptations threaten, you now have more than one tactic to carry you through on the path that God intends for your family.

Lord, thank You for guiding our family along our journey
and for giving us the strength to come so far.
Help us as we learn to become more active as a family.
Remind us daily to play together!
Instruct us as we apply our newfound knowledge and tools
so that we might keep going even during difficult times.
And, Father, please bless these precious children.
Amen.

Dear brothers and sisters, when troubles come
your way, let it be an opportunity for joy.
For when your faith is tested, your endurance
has a chance to grow.
So let it grow, for when your endurance is
fully developed, you will be strong in character
and ready for anything.

JAMES 1:2-4

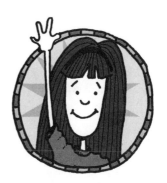

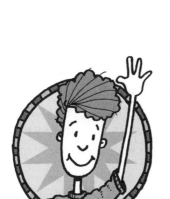

Chapter 8

MAKING IT WORK

Practical Ways to Connect with Your Child

You can't see it. You can't touch it.
Few say they have plenty of it.
Some say they don't have any of it.
You can invest it, spend it or save it.
You can prioritize it or you can fritter it away.
Some of us have too much of it on our hands.
Many of us feel we never have enough of it.
The way you use it can affect those you love.
It is time.

Time is such a valuable commodity, especially when it comes to our children. We *know* that the time we have with our children is very short. In 20 years, we won't recall our bank account balance or how clean our house was during these times, but the memories of those early words or the first scraped knee will be indelibly printed on our minds!

Of course, when the day is long and hard, time doesn't seem short enough! Jennifer laments, "Today the baby had the flu, the dog pooped in the living room, the twins bickered nonstop, and the hot water heater blew up and flooded the laundry room. Now that the kids are *finally* asleep, I just want to take a shower and finally have some *me* time!"

Time is funny that way—the moments we want to savor seem to fly by with a blink of an eye, while the challenges seem to drag on and on.

In light of the hectic demands of real life, you might wonder how on earth you can possibly find time to implement the suggestions in this book. You may think, *Are the authors from another planet?* Well, no— we aren't. In fact, we *do* know what it's like to be frazzled after a trying day. We also understand that, for many, lack of time can lead us to throw good intentions out the window and give up. And that the chaos of daily living sometimes tempts some of us to grab onto a quick fix in our desperate attempt to help our overweight child slim down.

Each of us has 10,080 minutes in every week of life—yet we often spend them in less than memorable ways. As we run to and fro, working and volunteering and running our "taxi service," it is so easy for our kids to get lost in the shuffle. God has blessed you with an awesome gift that is greater than anything else the world can offer: *your child*. We want to extend an invitation: Capture and savor each moment with this precious gift from God.

A busy dad shared his story with us. We hope that it inspires you.

We moved out to the country three years ago, and each time we head to town for shopping or appointments, we meander through a beautiful canyon and cross a bridge over the American River. The kids often beg to stop at the river to play, but I usually find a reason to say no. One dazzling summer morning, I asked myself what *really* was the problem with saying yes. I couldn't think of a single good reason, so I shocked us all by pulling over! The kids were giddy with excitement as we scampered down the path to a sandy beach along the river. I had the opportunity to pass on to my kids what my dad shared with me decades before—how to skip rocks. The kids' laughter and joy as the stones danced over the calm surface of the water was priceless! The whole experience taught me a valuable lesson: It doesn't take much time to reap rich rewards. The rest of the day they kept thanking me for what seemed a simple thing but meant the world to them.

We want to help you connect with your child and to savor every sacred moment. We all feel pushed to our limits at times, and we often can't figure out how to make positive changes and still get everything done. And yet, as you build a bridge with your child through your actions and words, we believe that the impossible will begin to feel doable. So, let's get started!

Connect Through Your Actions

Sometimes, it can take only a moment to connect with our kids. A shared look or a quick whispered compliment can let them know you are crazy about them. One dad admits: "I was as excited as Brian about the new Hot Wheels racing track he got for his birthday. I felt like a kid again as we raced against each other! He was pretty surprised to learn that I played with Hot Wheels when *I* was a kid."

It has been said that to find out what is really important to someone, you only need to look at his checkbook and his calendar. The truth is, we make time for the things that are important to us. We manage to carve out time for such things as watching TV, reading the newspaper each morning, surfing the Internet, talking on the phone, cleaning the house or taking a brisk walk around the neighborhood. So let's transform our family life by setting aside more of those 10,080 minutes to devote to the people we love. Take a few minutes at breakfast to put down the paper and talk with your son about his upcoming day. Shut down the computer in the evening and share devotions as a family. Through these small but powerful investments, your children will learn that they are extremely important.

Enjoying your child is like building a bridge, strengthening the connection from your heart to hers. Without a relationship built on trust, love *and* time, it is much more difficult to communicate with your child about important life issues. So start today to find ways to build that bridge!

Five-Minute Fun Fest

One family with a rather hectic schedule (like most of us!) invented a creative way of enjoying one other. "Family Couch Time" is a "cuddle fest" that spurs laughter and family bonding. Even their teenagers join in on the fun! The cuddle fest only lasts a few minutes, but the memories and the love being shared will last a lifetime.

In just five minutes each day, you and your child can:

- Toss a ball around
- Braid hair
- Draw a picture for Grandma
- Sit down for an old-fashioned cuddle fest
- Sing a song together
- Make a mud pie
- Play in the snow

- Play Tic-Tac-Toe
- Act out a famous nursery rhyme together ("Three Little Pigs" is fun!)
- Groom the dog
- Transplant flowers
- Look at the night sky
- Cut out a paper snow flake
- Make friendship bracelets out of string or yarn
- Color in a coloring book
- Give a back rub or a foot massage

If you don't typically do these things with your kids, the minute you say, "Wanna play Frisbee?" they might look at you as if you had just grown a third eyeball. That's okay! Get silly and be persuasive. Just tell them that if they don't play Frisbee, you will keep doing your Kermit the Frog imitation all day long until they change their minds. That should work!

In the space below, list some inventive five-minute activities you can do with your child during the next week.

_____

_____

_____

_____

_____

_____

_____

_____

_____

_____

_____

_____

_____

_____

_____

Joyful Journey

We spend *lots* of time in the car! So, make the most of time spent chauffeuring your kids from one activity to another. Use these "time tidbits" to connect with them and have some fun. Play the alphabet animal game: One person names an *A* animal. The next person identifies an animal whose name starts with *B* and so on, until you get to the end of the alphabet.

Or try the alphabet family game. Never heard of it? Well, you focus on one member of the family, and for every letter of the alphabet, everyone else thinks of a positive trait that describes that person. "*A* is for *amazing*—Daniel is amazing!" "*B* is for *brave*. He's brave, too!" Continue through the alphabet. On long rides, every family member can have a chance to be the focus of this positive and uplifting game.

Share prayer requests and pray for each other. The kids may ask for prayer for their friend's cousin's cat or for a favorite stuffed animal, but eventually, as they begin to feel comfortable and secure, they will share more personal needs. Don't hesitate to make prayer requests of your own with your children, as is appropriate for their age. Reassure them that you won't pray with your eyes closed while you are driving!

On family vacations, allow time for individualized activities in the car, while also letting the kids know what the game plan is. For instance, you could say, "At 3:30 we will have some family time!" As you drive, you can play old standard games like I Spy with My Little Eye or the license plate game, which involves writing down the names of every state license you see.

Take an audio recorder or camcorder on your road trip, and then give everyone a turn to record what happens en route to your destination. In their best broadcaster voice, they state the date and time, as well as your family's current location, then narrate details they want to add about the journey. Get really silly or elaborate as you interview one another! After you return home, play the tape or DVD and be entertained while reliving memories from your trip!

To encourage conversation, ask questions that everyone can answer—even Mom and Dad. Here are some starter suggestions.

- What was your best school day ever and why?
- What is the most memorable dream you have had?
- What was your favorite birthday ever and why?
- What was your favorite vacation and why?
- Tell us about your most embarrassing moment.
- When were you afraid? What did you do about it?

Have fun! Laugh together! Times such as these will bring everyone closer. This kind of bonding not only develops great memories, but also builds bridges on which you can depend when weightier matters need to be resolved.

Lingering Longer

With a little creativity and commitment, you can plan opportunities to linger longer with your children. Heading outside to throw baseball, spending an afternoon doing crafts or going on a shopping spree can be priceless time spent one on one with your child. Even if the budget is tight, you can go window-shopping together at the mall, as you both imagine how you would splurge on one another if you had a million bucks! Or sign up to take a class or play a team sport together. One daughter asked her mom if they could join a recreational softball league together—and Mom did it. What a great idea!

Marianne developed a regular habit of taking her daughter on a "girls' night out," beginning when Kami was only four years old. We hope her story inspires you!

At first we just went out and had fun together—trying on silly hats at the mall or having a picnic at a nearby playground. But, over the years, our girls' night out turned into an important time of sharing whatever was on her mind. Her first important questions about God, friends and boys all came during our girls' night out. She learned that she could ask me anything during these special times together . . . and could usually talk me into buying some new clothes or earrings! Now that she's almost a teenager, I've learned it is one of the few times that I have her undivided attention! I had no idea, years ago, what an important tradition we were building together.

Talk about bridge building!

List some outing or activity ideas that will allow you to intentionally spend quality time with your child:

_____

_____

_____

_____

_____

_____

_____

_____

_____

_____

_____

_____

Connect Through Your Words

Time invested in our kids often speaks louder than words, but words are powerful, too. You might confess to your daughter that you are absolutely crazy about her or announce to your son you are glad God made you his daddy. First Thessalonians 5:11 reminds us to encourage and build each other up. Often, if we don't intentionally speak kind, encouraging words, we end up nagging, criticizing and whining. In the end, we send our children messages that we never intended.

Michael is a successful professional in his mid-40s. He is tall, slim and the picture of health. He explains:

> All my life, my relatives told me I would be fat. My parents and most of my extended family were very overweight and I vividly recall being told that being fat was "in my genes." They joked

that I should "enjoy being thin while it lasts" because I would eventually be fat like everyone else. I've spent my entire life feeling fat . . . even though I never was. To this day, I have difficulty enjoying food due to the fear that I will eventually be overweight. Now that I'm a father myself, I try to remember to speak words to my daughter that will build her up rather than tear her down.

Michael's relatives may have wanted to be helpful or perhaps were enjoying what they thought was "harmless fun." However, their words were far from harmless. What children hear can become indelibly imprinted in their minds. Few parents ever intentionally say harmful things to their children, but even words that seem trivial or innocent can last a lifetime. So choose your words carefully—develop the habit of thinking before you speak.

The Word Wand

Do you ever wish you could snatch back your words before they reached someone's ears? Have you ever exploded and then realized that you sounded just like your mother? *Yikes!* The Word Wand will help in such situations.

Children are "whole body" listeners. When we speak, they take in *everything*—the expression on our face, the tone of our voice and our body language. "I love you" can easily become "Mom loves me, but she thinks I'm a failure" if we've said those words with disappointment written all over our face. Our emotional state often makes such an impact on our kids that they may not even hear our words. This is the reason that children so often fail the "What did I just say to you?" test.

Suzanne had been ill with the flu for several days when her youngest child developed an ear infection. She had missed two days of work, was behind on an important project and had been up most of the night with her sick baby. Her house was a mess. Walking into her oldest daughter's room, she discovered it was a complete wreck, topped off with an empty pizza box on the floor.

Suzanne's emotions reached the boiling point. "Lauren, I cannot *believe* that you ate the *entire* pizza! Don't you care *anything* about your health?! Stop staring at that stupid computer, and clean up this pig-sty you call a room. And if I *ever* catch you eating that much pizza again, I'll never buy another pizza as long as you live! Do you understand me? What did I just say?"

Her daughter, Lauren, responded with a blank stare, and she finally stuttered out a few words, "Uh, pizza . . . clean room . . . computer?" However, if Lauren had been completely honest, her answer might have been: "You said I'm a lazy, fat slob—and you don't like me very much." Suzanne, exhausted and overwhelmed by all the responsibilities crashing down upon her, was concerned for Lauren's health. But, instead of communicating *those* feelings, she lashed out at her. Lauren received a message completely different from what her mother had intended. It doesn't take much to hurt the very sensitive hearts of our children, and what can sometimes injure them most is the indiscriminate use of our tongue.

Take heart! We *can* move beyond our very human tendency to speak before we think. It starts with recognizing what our hearts *want* to say and finding ways to get *that* message across to our kids, rather than the stinging darts we often shoot in their direction. This is where the Word Wand comes in handy, as it helps us reflect on our words by examining four important aspects of communication:

1. What I thought and felt
2. What I said
3. What my child may have heard (based on my tone of voice, attitude and words)
4. What I could have said

As parents, we *mean* well. However, the way we communicate distorts the feelings of our heart to the point that the messages our child receives aren't accurate or recognizable.

After reading the following examples of the Word Wand—which pertain specifically to eating habits—you have an opportunity to make some entries of your own.

What I Thought and Felt	What I Said	What My Child May Have Heard and Thought	What I Should Have Said
My child is reaching for her third biscuit! I just put the plate out a couple of minutes ago. She eats food faster than I can dish it out! How will she ever lose weight? I must be a failure as a parent. I don't even cook healthy meals as I should, like other mothers I know.	"Put that biscuit back! You are eating like a pig! Stop cramming your food down so fast! You'll never fit into those new clothes if you keep eating that way!"	*Oh, my gosh! Mom just called me a pig! Everyone hates pigs because they are fat and smelly and gross. Now everyone is staring at me—I'm so embarrassed. I'll look awful in my new clothes. Next time I'll sneak some biscuits up to my room and eat them all by myself.*	"Honey, your mouth and stomach don't like to be crowded, and it takes a few minutes for your stomach to realize you're getting full. Slow down a little so that you can taste and enjoy what you're eating. Then your stomach will have a chance to let you know if it's getting full. I didn't do a very good job tonight of providing a variety of healthy food choices, so let's make sure we eat the right amounts, okay?"
There's an empty box of cookies on the floor. My child	"You've eaten an entire box of cookies? What on*	*Boy, I've really screwed up this time. I don't even*	"Honey, when you watch TV and eat at the same time,

must have eaten the whole thing during that TV show!	earth do you think you are doing?"	*remember eating the cookies, but no way will Mom believe that. I am such an idiot!*	you can't hear what your stomach is saying. Most people will eat more than they really need when watching TV. Next time, let's turn off the TV and eat at the table, okay?"
My child is obviously upset about something. She is gobbling down that pizza so fast she can't possibly taste it.	"Why are you stuffing your face full of pizza? Don't you realize that's why you are overweight?"	*I've had a terrible day, and now Mom has to remind me of how fat I am. I just can't get a break.*	"You seem to be upset. Let's go for a walk and talk about it."

Beginning with the left-hand column and then moving to the right, fill in a chart of your own using real-life or hypothetical situations. Let your thoughts flow freely as you fill out each column.

What I Said	What I Thought and Felt	What My Child May Have Heard and Thought	What I Should Have Said

Usually it takes some reflection, patience and prayer before we can recognize our own feelings, much less how best to communicate them. Sadly, our good intentions can evaporate in a moment of frustration, and thoughtless words can fly out of our mouths, taking on a life of their own! Communicating in a positive, effective manner has never been an easy task. Read what the apostle James has to say regarding the effect of our words:

> A word out of your mouth may seem of no account, but it can accomplish nearly anything—or destroy it! A careless or wrongly placed word out of your mouth can do that. By our speech we can ruin the world, turn harmony to chaos, throw mud on a reputation, send the whole world up in smoke and go up in smoke with it, smoke right from the pit of hell. With our tongues we bless God our Father; with the same tongues we curse the very men and women he made in his image. Curses and blessings out of the same mouth! (Jas. 3:5-6,9-10, *THE MESSAGE*).

Those are some pretty tough words. How often is our communication with our kids polluted with critical or harsh words? Then we are surprised that our children don't appear uplifted by our "wisdom"!

You can improve your "kid communication" skills by talking to your child right after you blow it and asking for forgiveness. Children often assume that they are at fault, even though they almost never say so. Even if you think it is obvious that *you* lost your cool and acted like an idiot, your child may still believe that *he* was responsible for your outburst, unless you tell him otherwise.

Spirit Moment: Humility

Carly's story speaks of a powerful character trait that is vital in parenting: humility.

> When my husband and I decided to have kids, I had very mixed emotions. My upbringing was far from ideal and I felt completely inadequate, knowing that I needed skills and abilities I didn't possess. Thank God for my husband. While Don didn't have the most ideal upbringing either, he is a humble man. I will never forget the first time I heard him pray with our two-year-old son, Christian. "Lord, I confess to You that I got really mad when Christian scribbled on the wall. Please forgive me for being so angry, Lord, and help me to be a better daddy." Then he said to Christian, "While you were wrong for scribbling on the walls, I should *never* lose my temper like that. Will you please forgive me for being so angry?"
>
> I was floored. In that moment I realized that my father had never once apologized to me for anything, even when he'd spanked me for something he later discovered I *hadn't* done! I learned from my husband that I needed to be humble enough to admit my mistakes, and let my children see me confess my sin to the Lord in prayer as well. Now when I'm impatient with my kids, I let them know that I was wrong and ask for their forgiveness. I really believe that this willingness to be humble is largely responsible for the great relationship that I enjoy with my 12- and 14-year-old kids.

Admitting we are wrong is hard, isn't it? But when we've messed up, make no mistake: God knows it, we know it, and our children know it. We lose nothing and gain everything when we humbly confess our imperfections and seek forgiveness.

Remember Suzanne, the end-of-her-rope mom who yelled at her daughter Lauren? Well, Suzanne later realized that she had completely blown it, so she had a heart-to-heart talk with her daughter and told her how overwhelmed she'd felt with her illness and that of the baby. Suzanne confessed that she didn't have the energy to help Lauren with her homework or even to remind her about keeping her room clean. Suzanne then admitted that she tends to turn to food rather than to God whenever she feels upset; she explained that the sight of the empty pizza box made her fear that Lauren was following in her footsteps—and that sent her over the edge.

Suzanne asked Lauren to forgive her for not trusting that God would take care of the family during difficult times, and she apologized for taking her frustrations out on her. She reaffirmed how much she loved Lauren and warmly expressed her appreciation for her beautiful, very responsible daughter. Lastly, she promised to communicate better in the future so that they could talk about their concerns without yelling. Lauren gave her mom a big hug and admitted she, too, tends to eat when she is upset. She promised that she would talk to her mom about her feelings the next time something was bothering her. Suzanne's humility paved the way for Lauren to feel safe enough to be vulnerable about her own struggle with emotional eating.

If communication with your children isn't working, consider possible reasons why. Think and pray about your responses, and then 'fess up and admit that you have been wrong when you've been overly critical or out of control. Ask for forgiveness, if needed, and discuss with your child how you might have handled things in a better way. You will be amazed at how your child will respond to this honesty, and it will help both of you the next time a similar situation occurs.

Building Bridges Through Affirmation

Affirmation is an important tool that fosters connection between family members. Yet how often do we affirm each other? Instead, we spend so much time within our family walls instructing or correcting: "Don't forget to take out the garbage!" "Have you finished your homework?" "You aren't leaving this house dressed like that!" Affirmation can be a breath of fresh air that transforms "Mealtime Madness" to "Mealtime Magnificence!" All it takes is a little creative planning and a heart tender to the leading of God's Spirit.

Playing the dinnertime Affirmation Game is a great place to start. Everyone draws another family member's name from a hat. Then, beginning with the adults, take turns affirming a character quality or skill of the person whose name was drawn. For instance, Mom drew John's name and said to him, "I admire the way I can trust you to be honest. Your word is good and you don't bend the truth. I appreciate and admire that character trait about you."

Here are some possible affirmations that could be offered by one sibling to another:

- "I like how neat you keep your stuff. I wish I could keep my stuff so clean!"

- "You're an amazing artist. That picture you drew last week of a horse was great!"

- "You always make me laugh. I really think you're funny. I like that about you."

- "You're such an incredible athlete. You're fast and a good sport."

- "You're such a fast reader. I would never have imagined anyone could read the books you do and in such a short time, too."

- "Yesterday when Jeff yelled at you, you stayed so calm. You have a lot of patience."

Obviously, it may take some time for kids to get the hang of this. Praise their good attempts, and gently help them see the difference between thanking someone for doing something and genuinely affirming who they are. As families learn to offer affirmations during mealtime (perhaps once each week, or more often if you like), they may find that the language of affirmation becomes a natural part of their everyday interactions with each other.

Below, list affirmations you can offer to each member of your family:

Family member _____
Affirmation:

_____

_____.

Family member _____
Affirmation:

_____

_____.

Family member _____
Affirmation:

_____

_____.

Family member _____
Affirmation:

_____

_____.

Attitude of Gratitude

Another important tool for fostering the positive use of words is through the expression of thankfulness. At mealtime, or some other time when the family is together in one place, ask family members to share something for which they are thankful. You might even develop different themes so that one evening everyone shares something about work or school for which he or she is thankful. Another session might involve thankfulness for family members or friends. This attitude of gratitude will foster dynamite exchanges and elicit observations about God's blessings—and you don't have to wait until Thanksgiving to do it!

Connect Through Problem-Solving

At this point in our journey, you've worked hard to take in new information, implement changes and enjoy new activities together. Hopefully, you're recognizing that your child is eating from "0 to 5" and enjoying Whole-Body Pleasers, even as you work on ways to develop a heart connection together. But maybe at this point you're wondering, *After all this time and all these changes, why doesn't he look different? I thought he would have lost weight by now!*

If the fire department ever visited your child's school, you're probably familiar with the phrase, "Stop, drop and roll." Let's modify this saying to help us identify mistakes and make positive corrections.

Ideally, your child will learn to be a fit kid in the same way she learned about money, manners or how to ride a bike. When she first fell off her bike, what worked best for getting her going again? Screaming? Manipulating? Overreacting rarely helps our kids learn from their mistakes. This is true whether playing soccer, riding a bike, or thinking and acting like a fit kid. If we blow up, whine or manipulate, especially at meal times, our kids get the message that this is a *really* big problem! And then food and eating issues become much tougher to handle. This tool will help you keep a cooler head and a warmer heart as you course correct. Now, when she fails to eat nutritious foods or exercise, you will be offering that encouragement and guidance that you offered when she fell off her bike. Your response will be, "Oh, shucks. We didn't do so well that time. Let's see if we can do better next time!"

Stop
When something goes wrong, *stop* and look with your eyes, but also with your heart. Take a moment and ask for God's insight and wisdom.

For instance, if your child ate when he wasn't hungry, is there something bothering him? What is his expression and demeanor? Did he use food to get attention or to "stuff down" frustration due to something that happened at school?

Did the Tummy Keys get forgotten? Can you use the Word Wand to see where a mistake may have occurred? Did you blow it? Do you need to ask his forgiveness? Perhaps you didn't plan well or were at your wits' end and simply threw up your hands and gave up. If the mistake was mostly your child's, what precipitated it? Was it an innocent mistake or more deliberate rebellion? Prayerfully evaluate what caused the temporary setback. Once you get into the habit of objectively examining rough spots in the road, effective course correction will become second nature.

Drop

Drop anything that hinders progress, such as emotional baggage. Avoid the temptation to play the blame game or to keep score. Instead, consider the situation from a detached, objective standpoint. This is a way of life, not a diet, so your child's success *today* is far less important than the long-term habits that are being cultivated. Keeping a great attitude is invaluable!

Are there habits and behaviors to change? An empty cookie bag on the floor might be a clue not to buy those cookies for a while or to put all snack foods out of sight so that no one is tempted. Maybe your child ate far more than she needed because you and your spouse were arguing at the table. If so, "drop" pride and ask for forgiveness; then resolve to make wiser choices the next time a similar situation arises. This models a humble heart for your child and makes you an emotionally safe person. Mistakes are opportunities to make better decisions in the future. Don't dwell on them.

Finally, *drop* to your knees. Whatever the issue is, lay it at Jesus' feet. Pour your heart out to Him and, before you know it, your perspective will change dramatically. Consider the words of Paul in his letter to the Philippians: "Don't worry about anything; instead, pray about everything. Tell God what you need, and thank him for all he has done. If you do this, you will experience God's peace, which is far more wonderful than the human mind can understand. His peace will guard your hearts and minds as you live in Christ Jesus" (Phil. 4:6-7).

Roll

Once you have a plan of action, *move on!* Let the past be the past. Fix your eyes on what is yet ahead! With a plan of action for the next time you face this situation, you are now good to go. Dwelling on past mistakes accomplishes nothing. Put the experience in your learning bank and forge ahead. Each moment matters. Recapture the spirit of discovery and adventure!

As Paul writes, "Since God chose you to be the holy people he loves, you must clothe yourselves with tenderhearted mercy, kindness, humility, gentleness, and patience. You must make allowance for each other's faults, and forgive the person who offends you. Remember, the Lord forgave you, so you must forgive others. And the most important piece of clothing you must wear is love. Love is what binds us all together in perfect harmony" (Col. 3:12-14).

No Simple Formulas

As we reflect on ways to connect with our children, we at times feel so inadequate, as though we were staring at our children from across the Grand Canyon. How often do we harbor regret over the harsh words we have used toward our children? How many times do we plan a day of fun and bonding, only to allow ourselves to be distracted by other responsibilities? How frequently are our good intentions ruined by anger and conflict?

There are no simple formulas to connecting with and loving our children. And yet, our God is able and willing to guide us on this path that is sometimes treacherous but that leads to unimaginable fulfillment. Your love *can* build a bridge to the heart of your child, spanning the broadest chasm. It is our hope and prayer that you will seek God's face, search for His wisdom, accept His grace and experience His love.

Lord, please bless our heartfelt effort to do the right thing
for our children and forgive us our shortcomings.
Help us learn to connect with our children so that
they may understand the depth of our love for them.
Reveal to us any harmful words or attitudes that need to be changed.
As we stumble along this parenting path,
please use our failures and successes to draw our children toward You.
Thank You for the honor of raising these amazing children,
and help us to savor each moment and store them in our hearts forever.
Amen.

And now these three remain:
faith, hope and love.
But the greatest of these is love.
1 CORINTHIANS 13:13, *NIV*

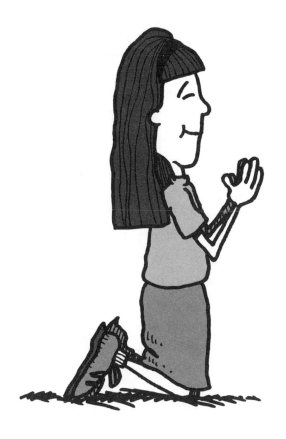

CHAPTER 9

HUNGRY HEARTS

Recognizing the Inner Needs of Your Child

Christmas lights dance on the tree. Torn paper and ribbons are strewn about. The puppy frolics amongst all the new toys and empty boxes, having her way with the tissue paper. Surrounded by numerous gadgets and gizmos, Jordan tears open a brightly colored package and pulls out an RC monster truck! He raises his arms in the air, shouting with glee, *"Yes! It's just what I asked for!"* Suddenly he glances around frantically and then dives under the tree. He scrambles on his tummy, flattens every bulge and bump, and even peeks under the tree skirt, his eyes filled with hope. With a heavy sigh, Jordan turns to his dad, seeking adult confirmation of what his search has concluded, *"Is that all there is?"*

Most of can identify with the "Is that all there is?" attitude. Whether it is the anticipated promotion at work, the next TV (with a bigger, flatter screen), or the latest iPod (now able to store TV shows, games, movies and more songs than ever before!), adults and kids alike have a seemingly insatiable appetite for *more.* Toy boxes are never big enough, closets are always bulging, and our garages are overflowing with "stuff."

Among the tons of toys that kids play with, one favorite for many young children is a "shape sorter"—a small table or box with wooden cut-outs of different shapes, such as squares, circles and triangles. Blocks in corresponding shapes are designed to fit through various holes. Toddlers spend *hours* trying to force a square block into the round hole. They shove, grunt, push harder—and finally throw the uncooperative block across the room! As parents, we hand them the correct shape, then patiently watch their fierce determination as those tiny hands work to get it into the one spot where it fits perfectly. Finally, shining eyes and gleeful giggles announce their proud victory!

In fact, our hearts—and those of our children—are a lot like those shape sorters, and the holes represent the inner longings of our hearts. Kids have such a fun, happy-go-lucky demeanor, and they are *so darn cute!* When we hear those giggles and watch that bundle of energy go zooming by, it is sometimes easy for us to forget that our children have cares or worries. The truth is, *they do!* They feel anxious about being accepted by others, they get their feelings hurt by a friend who chooses someone else, or have their hearts crushed by a boy who doesn't know they exist. They desperately long to hit the ball out of the park, to receive high-fives and admiration from others, or to hear an enthusiastic "Way to go, buddy!" from Dad.

Today, we are going to look more closely at those "holes in the heart"—the inner longings of your child. During this special time together, we invite you to pour your heart out to God and ask Him to reveal any areas in your child's life in which there may be some hidden, unmet needs.

A Hungry Heart

When Debbie asked her friend Heather to tell her about the Fit Kids method, Heather explained, "One part of this approach is helping the kids learn to eat only when they are hungry."

"Hmm, eat when hungry?" Debbie responded. "What a novel idea!"

Why don't we all do this naturally? If we aren't physically hungry, then *why* do we eat? As we said earlier, often we're just trying to jam something—food in this case—into the hole in our hearts. Our "hungry hearts" insist on being filled. Let us illustrate how this works.

On arriving home after school one day, Alyssa plunged headfirst into a bag of potato chips. Her mom walked into the TV room and asked, "Sweetheart, are you hungry?" Alyssa looked up and mumbled, "I guess not." Having built a relationship of trust and love, her mom sat down next to Alyssa and kindly inquired, "What's up, sweetie?" Alyssa's eyes welled up with tears. "I guess, well . . . I'm lonely," she said softly.

Alyssa had turned to food to numb her pain, thinking she could make the afternoon more bearable by sharing it with a bag of chips. The truth is, if she had kept eating and emptied the entire bag, Alyssa would have been stuffed and uncomfortable, but her loneliness would have remained. She attempted to shove a square-shaped block into a round hole, and it just didn't work! In fact, without the timely intervention of her mother, the guilt of her inappropriate eating might easily have resulted in further isolation.

Frequently, our children think they really *are* hungry when something deeper is going on. There *was* something within Alyssa crying to be recognized, acknowledged and satisfied, and to ignore or minimize this inner hunger is a missed opportunity. What a gift we give our kids when we teach them how to distinguish between stomach hunger and heart hunger. After all, we know the answer to the underlying deeply felt need!

Adults are certainly not immune from the appeal of emotional eating. David relates his story:

> I will never forget how I felt while waiting for my medical college entrance test scores. On the day of reckoning, I was so nervous that I bought a cheesecake and ate half of it *all by myself*. Later that day I received my test scores and they were great—much better than I had dared to hope. I was so excited that I ate the rest of the cheesecake to celebrate! Afterward, I felt like a fool. I was too embarrassed to tell even my wife about it.

David's nervousness, insecurity and concern over whether his dreams would be realized seemed to justify turning to cheesecake to help him bear the burden. Then the sudden elation of "Yes! I did it!" led him to celebrate with the same food that had "shared" his misery. But the end result was shame rather than celebration. Shame often sends us into the darkness—hiding, sneaking, often distancing ourselves from God—and it can even lead to addictive behavior. Sometimes, like David, we think we can make food fit the shape of any hole within our hearts! But the truth is, food simply doesn't deliver what we really need.

Sometimes it is tough to identify an emotion that is prompting us to grab for the cookies when we aren't hungry. We may eat from boredom or habit. Occasionally a certain person or a particular setting may trigger a desire for food.

Don planned a home movie night with his family. He gathered the provisions for the evening—sodas, popcorn and cookies—and then eagerly assembled a big pan of nachos to stick in the oven. As the kids gathered around the TV, it struck Don that he wasn't even hungry! He had just been operating on auto pilot. He confessed, "I suddenly realized that I just naturally associated family nights with a 'food fest'!

The kids looked at me with baffled expressions and wondered what had happened to our plan to pursue wise choices and eat only when hungry. Boy, were they right!"

When going along with the crowd at a family gathering, church potluck or movie night, we may not think through the choices we make. In moments like these, something other than physical hunger often drives the urge to eat. We can help our children to see the truth about such behavior by teaching them to ask themselves, "What's up? *Why* am I grabbing for the food?"

Some Common Needs

Have you noticed situations in which your child eats when he isn't hungry? While specific scenarios are different for everyone, attempting to answer our deeper needs with food, things or popularity is like slapping a Band-Aid on an internal hemorrhage. Let's turn our focus to some of the common needs of children and see how to point them away from cheap substitutes and toward the One who can really meet those needs.

The Need for Security

Do you remember the first time you left your child with a grandparent for that much-needed weekend getaway? Can you recall her first day of school? Chances are, the way she reacted to those situations was driven by a single inward question: "Will I be cared for?" When you returned from the weekend with gifts, stories, hugs and kisses, her inner insecurities disappeared—she knew she was loved. As she craned her neck at the end of the school day, searching for your car, the relief in her little body when she spotted you could be seen from miles away!

One of the earliest and deepest needs of infants is for security. While they require being fed and clothed, their *deepest* longing—one that keeps parents up at all hours of the day and night—is to be cared for. A consistent response to their cries satisfies the longing in their little hearts for security.

As children grow and develop, the need for security intensifies. Sometimes children feel insecure because of their emotional makeup, a stressful past or a specific trauma. Perhaps Dad used to leave the house every morning, plant a kiss on Jason's cheek and say, "I'll see you tonight, buddy"—and then one evening Dad didn't return. Or a fourth-grader doesn't have clean clothes and is embarrassed because she looks different from everyone else at school.

Rather than merely reacting to the behaviors that cause you concern, evaluate *why* your kids are doing what they do and address whatever is beneath the surface. When children lack the security for which they long, they respond in a variety of ways. Some become overly responsible at a young age, carrying loads their young minds and hearts were never meant to bear. These stalwart soldiers might take on adult responsibilities, such as cooking, cleaning or taking care of younger children, in order for the family to appear "normal." Other children misbehave, overeat or engage in reckless behaviors involving drugs, sex or other counterfeits, hoping to find the security they are seeking or to convince themselves that they do *not* need anything—or anyone.

In spite of our best efforts, we sometimes find ourselves unable to keep a rising tide from coming in and changing the complexion of our home life. Death, divorce, loss of a job or a financial catastrophe can have a profound effect on any child. Please remember that God will *never* forsake you or your young one—there is no circumstance too hard for God and nothing beyond the reach of His mercy and grace. Turn to Him with any and every situation, and trust in Him to pull you through.

God intends to spin all our disappointments, failures and mistakes into gold. Being perfect just *isn't* part of the parenting job description, and God knows that we *all* fall short. Even Mary and Joseph, God's choice for Jesus' earthly parents, lost young Jesus during the Feast of Passover and didn't know where He was for three days! What a relief it is for our kids when we become transparent and admit our failures. Children will breathe a sigh of relief when they see our humanity, reassuring them that they don't have to be perfect and that our love for them is not based on performance.

God understands the high calling of parenting. Nothing can separate you or your children from the love of Jesus Christ—nothing you do, say, think or feel. God has answered the question "Will I be cared for?"

with a resounding "Yes!" His answer is, without a doubt, intended for both you *and* your child.

Bringing It Home

Take a moment to reflect on the condition of your home life. Chaotic living, isolation or frequent conflict can cause children to feel extremely insecure. On the other hand, a loving environment with clear boundaries your child can count on gives him the security he needs in order to thrive.

If you and your spouse are like two ships passing in the night, consider carving out a sacred few minutes each evening to sit on the couch and share what happened during the day. Be sure to explain to your children *in advance* that this is Mom and Dad's time. If your children resist this idea (as indeed they might at first), let them know that there will be family time afterward, which will include a big group hug. The amazing thing is, even 10 minutes spent alone with your spouse can make a huge difference! (More time is even better, of course!)

One couple discovered that this was indeed a powerful way of providing a sense of security for their young son, Stuart.

> With our busy schedules, we had unintentionally let time with each other slide. Stuart began having nightmares many nights, and we were concerned that there could be something wrong with him, as he had always been a good sleeper. One evening, we got a glimpse into his little heart when he asked, "If you get divorced, who will I live with?" We were shocked at his question, but we found, after some sharing time together, that another preschooler's parents were divorcing. He had witnessed our lack of time together and jumped to a painful conclusion.

They spent time that evening reassuring Stuart that they loved each other and were not divorcing. Then they apologized to each other and to their son for losing sight of their priorities. As they reestablished a nightly routine of evening time together, Stuart's nightmares quickly resolved.

Children are sometimes the "emotion monitors" for the entire family and may sense a problem even before their parents do. If your child is exhibiting inexplicable behaviors, consider whether tension or conflict in your marriage may be causing a sense of insecurity. Ask the Lord which security needs you can provide for your child, knowing that ultimately your child will experience her greatest sense of security from a personal relationship with God.

The Need to Belong
Babies cling to Mom and Dad, often to the exclusion of nearly everyone else. Preschool boys bond with other boys—no girls allowed! Older children foster deeper friendships with smaller circles of friends, promising to be "best friends forever." The social life of teenagers carries the highest priority as they establish their individual identity and explore romantic relationships, often turning to peers for support. Underlying all these stages are the family relationships, which hopefully provide a consistent sense of belonging throughout this maturing process.

This inner need for belonging and acceptance is the driving force in all relationships. If you need proof, you don't have to look far! Your daughter may sit next to her best friend each day at lunch, wear the same style clothes as her classmates or even speak in the exact same phrases as her friends. Your son may ask to grow his hair down to his shoulders, or shave it off entirely, depending on what his buddies are doing. Anything that makes a child stand out or that threatens his sense of belonging can be painful. At the same time, what might seem adorable or special to a parent, such as beautiful bright-red hair, a lovely singing voice or superior intelligence, can be a liability in a child's eyes if it sets her apart from her peers.

Megan recalls her childhood experience of being ostracized at school because she was extremely bright and excelled academically.

> God blessed me with intelligence and I truly am thankful for that, but I didn't always feel that way. I was moved a grade forward in school—gifted programs didn't exist back then—and was forever labeled as the "smart" kid or "the brain." My parents

didn't understand why it bothered me so and were critical of my lack of gratitude. But all I wanted at that time was to fit in with the other kids. *I just wanted to belong.*

Do you sense that your child feels he *doesn't* belong? Does he seem withdrawn or apathetic about playing with others? When he is interacting with other kids, does he seem awkward, withdrawn or aggressive? Isolating himself, hitting, kicking, biting or attention-gaining behaviors, such as showing off or becoming the class clown, are all clues that a child lacks a sense of belonging. To counter his sense of isolation, he may turn to the most readily available thing—food—in an attempt to soothe himself. As he gets older, he might turn to drugs, alcohol or sex, or join a group of friends that you don't approve of, simply in an effort to feel that he belongs.

If your child is acting out, put on your "heart goggles" and try to figure out what issues could be contributing to these behaviors. No matter how much you would like to meet *all* of your child's needs, a parent's influence is limited. Your child's ultimate need for acceptance is met through a personal relationship with God—the perfect Parent whose mercy, love and compassion are never-ending. Turn to Him for guidance, as you strive to understand the inner workings of your child's heart and mind.

Bringing It Home
Helping our children connect with others provides a much-needed sense of acceptance. Sometimes, their lack of belonging may even indicate a lack of connection at home. Consider whether there might be activities (see the previous chapter) that could help build a bridge between you and your child.

Charlie was concerned at his son's refusal to play on a baseball team, even though he was a very good player. "When we played in the backyard, Sam did great! He talked about baseball constantly and couldn't wait to play. But when it came time to join the other kids, he would hide behind me and never set foot on the field. Finally, I asked if it might help if I became an assistant coach. His eyes lit up like

Christmas trees!" For the remainder of the season, Sam headed out to the field next to Dad, with his head held high. Later in the season when Charlie was late to a game, Sam was already out on the field with the others. He had learned to interact with other kids, and he had also learned a valuable lesson about how important he was to his dad.

Darren, an autistic teenager, began to connect with others when he and his family volunteered to be greeters at their church. When Darren saw that he could make people smile as he welcomed them with a hug or handshake, he realized God had a place for him.

If your child balks at the notion of participating in the school play, perhaps she'd enjoy being a "junior assistant," helping to decorate the set instead. It's important that we help our children find a place in the larger world—a place that is a good fit for them.

The Need for Self-Worth

One of the deepest, most fundamental needs of children of *all* ages is the need to be validated—to feel that they matter. Little girls want to feel beautiful and captivating, longing to hear how lovely they are. Little boys desperately need to know that they measure up, especially in their father's eyes. Sadly, many men spend their entire lives fulfilling an angry father's pronouncement that "you'll never amount to anything!"

A parent's words and attitudes have a powerful impact on children. When Mom blurts, "I look so fat in this dress! If I don't spend every day in the gym next month, I'll just have to skip the party," her daughter begins to believe that beauty is skin-deep and that her worth is based on her appearance. Then Dad says, "Honey, I'll be home after bedtime again. I won't leave the office until I get this project right. If I don't finish it tonight, I won't get the big promotion." His son, overhearing this conversation, may begin to believe that "measuring up" means pleasing those who are in authority.

While we all want to raise our children to be successful, attractive, strong and well-mannered, our primary focus should never be to measure their success—or failure—by the world's standards. Instead, our sincere desire is to cultivate and nurture them so that they realize and fulfill the unique and special purpose that God intends for them.

Charles Swindoll relates the following story about artist Benjamin West:

> One day his mother went out, leaving him in charge of his lit-
> tle sister, Sally. In his mother's absence he discovered some
> bottles of colored ink and began to paint Sally's portrait. In
> doing so, he made a very considerable mess of things with ink
> blots all over. His mother came back. She saw the mess, but
> said nothing. She picked up the piece of paper and saw the
> drawing. "Why," she said, "it's Sally!" and she stooped to kiss
> him. Ever after Benjamin West used to say, "My mother's kiss
> made me a painter."[1]

God has a special plan for each and every child. It is important to identify and encourage areas of potential and assure our children they *do indeed matter*. After all, they hold a place of honor in our hearts far above their performance, appearance or social status.

Bringing It Home

One elementary school's program, called Caught Being Good!, was a rousing success. Each time a student was "caught" making a good choice, he received a special "buck" that could later be cashed in for various prizes. Let's take a similar approach: When our kids do something *good*, let's "catch them"—and tell them!

It is important to recognize and cultivate the unique gifts and passions God gave your child. Praise him for these positive attributes, but also be thankful for the "difficult" areas, which may represent special characteristics that God will gently mold and shape as only He can. As we spend more time connecting with our kids, we may be pleasantly surprised by some hidden attributes that we didn't even realize existed!

Ultimately, self-worth comes from having an understanding of who we are in Jesus Christ, who gave His life in exchange for our pardon. When we accept how precious we are to God, it is hard *not* to have a sense of self-worth. Share Bible verses with your child (in a translation that she can understand) to help her appreciate the value God has placed on each of us.

For we are God's masterpiece. He has created us anew in Christ
Jesus, so that we can do the good things he planned for us long
ago (Eph. 2:10).

You made my whole being; you formed me in my mother's body.
I praise you because you made me in an amazing and wonderful
way (Ps. 139:13-14, *NCV*).

The Need for Forgiveness

Most of us have known kids who are "good-choice challenged"! It is as
if trouble finds them like iron filings drawn to a magnet.

Consider the story of Lamont, who entered Cindy's first-grade
classroom after the school year was already under way. Sassy and disre-
spectful, he had a reputation for fighting, even though he was only seven years old. Cindy provided appropriate consequences for Lamont's
behavior, but she also extended forgiveness. She began having one-on-
one time with Lamont to teach him to read. She goes on to share the
rest of her story.

> I was fortunate that I had two classroom aids who could assist
> the other children while I spent some time each day with Lamont.
> He didn't know the alphabet yet, but he was quite bright and
> caught on quickly. With the time and attention I gave him, he
> flourished. I'll admit that, at times, it was hard to set aside all
> the "wrongdoing" for which he was known, but we focused on
> his willingness to be taught and, as he learned to read, he stopped
> fighting with other kids. He actually became one of the most
> delightful children in my entire first-grade class. I truly believe he
> blossomed because someone wasn't holding his wrongs against
> him, possibly for the first time in his young life. The anger that
> had characterized him just vanished.

Children need to know that the grownups in their lives will look
beyond their offenses to the possibilities ahead, and that regardless of
what they *do*, it's who they *are* that we love. We don't endorse turning a

blind eye to behavior that is inappropriate: Lamont was held accountable for his wrongdoings, but his good choices were joyfully celebrated. As God's Word says, "Love does not count up wrongs that have been done" (1 Cor. 13:5, *NCV*).

The need for forgiveness goes both ways, as Larissa wisely recognized.

> When I get angry, I sometimes tend to jump to conclusions before I have all the facts. Once when Samantha and Joey were playing together, all seemed to be going well until I heard a loud shriek, I ran into the living room and found both of them crying. Joey frequently gets too aggressive with his little sister, so when I found her on the floor, I automatically assumed it was his fault and punished him without getting all the information. When the truth finally tumbled out, it was clear that I had made a mistake. I went to both children and confessed I had been wrong, asking them to forgive me for jumping to conclusions.

Larissa's actions spoke volumes to her children, and the whole family was able to experience the sweet perfume of forgiveness.

No matter how mad or frustrated we get, or how much our kids break our hearts, they must be confident that we will always welcome them with open arms and forgiveness. Lacking this confidence, children will look elsewhere for unconditional love and forgiveness—only to find counterfeits, such as food. Or they may compound mistakes by "running and hiding" to avoid the expected criticism. As we strive to provide a safe environment in which children can admit they blew it and can ask for forgiveness, they will find relief and rest for the burdens they often carry.

Bringing It Home

One way to lead by example is to ask for forgiveness from your children when you know you have messed up, just as Larissa did. Let them hear the language of forgiveness from you, and they will be more likely to use it as well. By saying "I'm sorry" and asking, "Will you please forgive me?" you are admitting that you have wronged the other person in some way and are acknowledging that they can choose to release you through their forgiveness.

There is only One who will *never* let us down. He provides forgiveness for anything and everything, whenever we need it. He is the One who formed and fashioned us and knows our hearts intimately and personally. Having received God's grace, we know that forgiveness covers a multitude of sins—there is no ache or void that it cannot fill.

The Ultimate Heart Hunger

We wrote earlier about the holes that children have in their hearts, longing to be filled. As parents, we rightfully feel responsible for filling those holes as we address our child's inner longings. Yet according to Solomon, God has fashioned a *God-shaped* hole inside each human heart (see Eccles. 3:11). Rather than a square, triangle or circle, the only peg that will fit into our God-shaped hole is the God-shaped peg—the Lord Himself.

God longs to fill that empty place in our hearts, proving just how amazing He is! From the silly duck-billed platypus, to the intricate design of the peacock's tail, to the tallest Giant Sequoia trees, and to the thundering cascade of Niagara Falls, God has created every aspect of the world to demonstrate His creativity, glory and love.

Like the Mother Bunny in the classic book *The Runaway Bunny*, the Lord relentlessly pursues each one of us.

> Where can I go from your Spirit? Where can I flee from your presence? If I go up to the heavens, you are there; if I make my bed in the depths, you are there. If I rise on the wings of the dawn, if I settle on the far side of the sea, even there your hand will guide me, your right hand will hold me fast (Ps. 139:7-10, *NIV*).

Yet the strange thing is that we, like Baby Bunny, keep on running. And we keep stuffing that God-sized hole in our hearts with anything and everything *other* than that for which it was made. Like the toddler trying for all he's worth to fit a triangle block into the round hole, we try stuffing things like food, friends, electronic gizmos, popularity—or maybe even church activities—in order to fill that void.

Parents and kids alike experience failure and shame, as we continually fall down, then get up—and then fall down again! Is there a woman alive who cannot identify with Eve, unable to trust God with her heart, believing instead that she must take matters into her own hands? Doesn't every man recognize Adam's pain when, in the most important moment of his life, he stood passively to the side and denied his very nature? When these failures strike deep into our hearts, we long to stuff that hole with anything that might ease the pain. Rather than turning to the One who can fill the hole in our hearts, we may instead tend to hide or run away.

While children often represent rare slices of goodness and innocence, even *they* misbehave—in case you haven't noticed!

Faye asked her mischievous, freckle-faced son, "Justin, why did you hit your sister?" to which he responded with seemingly repentant, downcast eyes, "I don't know . . . I didn't mean to! I'm sorry, Mom." As Faye knelt down and hugged him, certain that his confession was sincere, Justin looked over her shoulder at his sister and stuck out his tongue.

Sometimes it is as if our children are performing a skit portraying Paul's very words:

I don't understand myself at all, for I really want to do what is right, but I don't do it. Instead, I do the very thing I hate . . . Oh, what a miserable person I am! (Rom. 7:15,24).

Each of us—adults and children alike—have an aching emptiness inside that leads to behaviors we don't understand. Try as we might, on our own we just cannot behave ourselves. We, like Justin, apologize with one breath and stick out our tongue a moment later! Nevertheless, out of His unfathomable love, the Creator of the universe humbled Himself and chose to come to us. Jesus came to extend forgiveness and to show us grace and truth so that we might know God and live with Him forever.

As we welcome the Lord into our lives, He will flood every hole, crack, crevice and empty place that exists within us. He alone is able to quench our thirst and satisfy our hunger.

How precious is your unfailing love, O God! All humanity finds shelter in the shadow of your wings. You feed them from the abundance of your own house, letting them drink from your rivers of delight. For you are the fountain of life, the light by which we see (Ps. 36:7-9).

By God's grace, this is the truth that we can model and teach our children, day by day. While our kids may learn important lessons in Sunday School or at other church activities, their most effective understanding of a living, breathing relationship with God comes from us. And, as we guide them, our own faith will be strengthened.

Annie relates a moving experience in her son's life—and in her own heart as well.

We've been taking Casey to church every Sunday since he was a baby. At one point, he began asking a million questions: "Why did Jesus die?" "Why didn't He just strike the bad people dead?" "What is sin?" "Does God see *everything* I do?" I found myself struggling for answers! After weeks and months of learning and growing together, Casey came to my room one night. "Mom, I've decided something. I want to believe in Jesus." After talking for a few minutes, my dear son prayed, "Jesus, I'm sorry for when I do wrong things—will You forgive me? Thanks that You forgive me no matter what I do. Since You love everybody, and never did anything wrong, and beat all the bad guys, and got raised up from the dead, I've decided to believe in You. Please take care of me. I want to grow up to be just like You and come to heaven to be with You and Grandma. Amen."

Oh, the joy that washes over our souls during moments like this! May we all experience such tender, innocent, childlike faith. And may we remember ourselves that Jesus calls each of us to respond with that same innocence and trust. As our children open their hearts and accept the One who created them in intimate detail, they gain the very keys to the Kingdom: "Jesus said, 'Let the children come to me. Don't stop them! For the Kingdom of Heaven belongs to such as these'" (Matt. 19:14).

Our highest calling as parents is *not* to solve *all* of our children's problems, but to direct them to the One who has all the answers.

Lord, thank You that You love us
and offer the solution to our heart's greatest need.
Please give us wisdom to know how best to encourage our children
to distinguish between heart hunger and stomach hunger.
Help us to give them the love, sense of security, belonging
and worth that are within our human power.
Above all, help us to point them to You.
We pray that they may know You, O Lord.
Amen.

And this is the way to have eternal life—
to know you, the only true God,
and Jesus Christ, the one you sent to earth.

JOHN 17:3, *NIV*

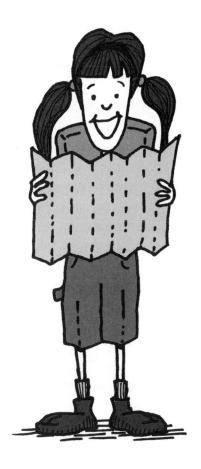

CHAPTER 10

OBSTACLE COURSE

Preparing for and Overcoming Challenges

Ellen's family was happy and healthy, seemingly without a care in the world. But one day, her husband arrived home with a bombshell.

Steve received a sudden job transfer, and before we knew it, we were packing to move to the other end of the country! Our family, friends, church and support structure were all left in the dust. It was such a shock that I'm afraid none of us reacted very well. As we attempted to settle into our new lives, we let important areas slide. We stopped exercising, began eating a lot of fast food and spent almost every evening parked in front of the TV. Our children seemed to gain weight overnight! Now we are dealing with all the same stress, plus the added pressure of two overweight children. I'd give *anything* to turn the clock back so that we could react reasonably to the changes.

From the mundane to the catastrophic, life's obstacles trip us up and threaten our success. To help prepare for such challenges, let's examine some of the common obstacles that you may encounter on the path to a fit and healthy life. This is truly where the rubber hits the road. Healthy habits are fairly manageable when life is rosy and calm, but when the storm clouds gather and let loose their fury, it's a different story entirely!

Max Lucado nails it perfectly in his rousing story of Chippie the parakeet:

The problems began when Chippie's owner decided to clean Chippie's cage with a vacuum cleaner. She removed the attachment from the end of the hose and stuck it in the cage. The phone rang, and she turned to pick it up. She'd barely said "hello" when "sssopp!" Chippie got sucked in.

The bird owner gasped, put down the phone, turned off the vacuum, and opened the bag. There was Chippie—still alive, but stunned.

Since the bird was covered with dust and soot, she grabbed him and raced to the bathroom, turned on the faucet, and held

Chippie under the running water. Then, realizing that Chippie was soaked and shivering, she did what any compassionate bird owner would do . . . she reached for the hair dryer and blasted the pet with hot air.

Poor Chippie never knew what hit him.

A few days after the trauma, the reporter who'd initially written about the event contacted Chippie's owner to see how the bird was recovering. "Well," she replied, "Chippie doesn't sing much anymore—he just sits and stares."

It's not hard to see why. Sucked in, washed up, and blown over . . . that's enough to steal the song from the stoutest heart.[1]

Do you ever feel a bit like Chippie? Raising your family as best you can, minding your own business, when suddenly—*bam!* Out of nowhere, the storm clouds hit and everything changes in an instant. You look around, wondering how you got here, thinking, *Who turned on the vacuum cleaner? How did I wind up under a cold faucet of water? Where did that giant blow dryer come from?*

When challenges strike, it is easy to forget everything you have learned about health and fitness. Somehow, consuming an entire bag of chocolate chip cookies under such circumstances seems justified!

How can we avoid such setbacks and derailments?

The person who trusts in the Lord will be blessed. The Lord will show him that he can be trusted. He will be strong, like a tree planted near water that sends its roots by a stream. It is not afraid when the days are hot; its leaves are always green. It does not worry in a year when no rain comes; it always produces fruit (Jer. 17:7-8, *NCV*).

Oh, to be like a tree, deeply planted by a life-giving stream—verdant, green, lush and fruitful, each and every day. The truth is, no matter how well grounded we may be, life is filled with hot, scorching seasons that often put us to the test and may cause us to wilt. We may face long periods of drought when we pray for rain. Just when we make positive changes and think we are on the right track, something unexpected hits us from the blind side. Before we can blink, our lives have been turned upside down and survival seems to be all that matters.

You can avoid setbacks and derailments when pursuing a healthier lifestyle by preparing for life's uncertainties. Knowing where to turn for ultimate strength, along with newfound knowledge and effective tools, can help you develop deep roots that sink into rich soil. As you draw nourishment and strength from God, you will be able to withstand sudden changes and difficult circumstances.

So let's get ready for whatever obstacles might be lurking around the corner.

The High Hurdle of the American Dream

The stress, anxiety and chaos of our lives can make fitness a low priority. We live in a fast-paced society surrounded by those who seek to *have* more and *do* more—and that makes it difficult to cultivate healthy habits. America has been blessed with prosperity beyond our wildest dreams. We, as a nation, have all we could possibly want—and more. And yet we continue to work harder, overspend, do more and enjoy less.

The prophet Jeremiah described the tree-like strength of those who trust in the Lord. But a few verses earlier, he described those who do *not* place their trust in Him. His words, uttered long ago, describe how many people in our culture live.

> Cursed is the strong one who depends on mere humans, who thinks he can make it on muscle alone and sets God aside as dead weight. He's like a tumbleweed on the prairie, out of touch with the good earth. He lives rootless and aimless in a land where nothing grows (Jer. 17:5-6, *THE MESSAGE*).

Do you sometimes feel as if your family is being tossed to and fro between deadlines, commitments and responsibilities? At times, we all feel this way. On Sundays we might drink in spiritual nourishment and leave church with a sense of purpose and faith, but from Monday through Saturday, we can lose our spiritual focus, our balance and, sadly, even our hope. Part of the reason may be because we are surrounded with those who want it all, and it is so easy to get sucked into believing that we must follow their path.

True joy doesn't come from outward success, but from within as we turn our hearts toward God. Today, are you willing to prayerfully examine the lifestyle of your family? Are you standing firm, sinking your roots deep into His soil, faithfully following the path God has laid out for you? Or have you been unexpectedly blindsided, feeling overwhelmed and wondering how you can possibly devote some sacred moments needed to raise a fit kid?

> Therefore we do not lose heart. Though outwardly we are wasting away, yet inwardly we are being renewed day by day. For our light and momentary troubles are achieving for us an eternal glory that far outweighs them all. So we fix our eyes not on what is seen, but on what is unseen. For what is seen is temporary, but what is unseen is eternal (2 Cor. 4:16-18, *NIV*).

As we scurry from place to place, our focus is often on the world around us—we act as if this life and these circumstances are permanent. But they aren't! Let's focus on what really matters!

As you stand in the starting blocks each day, gazing at the enormously tall hurdle that represents the American Dream, perhaps you might consider a new strategy. Instead of striving to make it over that hurdle, ask God for guidance for a different path altogether. Actively look for the narrow path that represents what God intends for you and your child. He will provide the direction, courage and strength needed to overcome all obstacles. "This is what the Lord says: 'Stand at the crossroads and look; ask for the ancient paths, ask where the good way is, and walk in it, and you will find rest for your souls' " (Jer. 6:16, *NIV*).

The Bumpy Road of Tradition and Habits

Another hurdle for us to overcome lies in the habits, traditions and sinfulness that are deeply ingrained in our lifestyle. Many of these result from our upbringing and remain embedded in our hearts and minds throughout our lives. These habits learned in childhood might impact when, what and how much you eat, without your even being aware of it. While some longstanding traditions are great to pass on to your children, others aren't necessarily the legacy you want to leave.

One example of such a tradition involves get-togethers for the Jennings family. Regardless of the occasion—weddings, holidays, reunions or weekend picnics—food is *always* front and center. In fact, one family member describes the omnipresence of food this way: "We are so used to eating together that if I see my sister, I automatically look for the food!"

Traditions are often borne out of good times, such as the love and fellowship that stem from family togetherness. However, it is easy to give food a higher priority than it deserves. Our children observe our behavior and draw unspoken cues from us, quickly learning that second helpings and extra desserts are a necessary part of any celebration.

Another similar situation may occur when family relationships or friendships generate tension or conflict. A common reaction is to turn to food as a way to get through the event. Consider the example of Melissa, who visits her father on the weekends.

> I love to spend time with my dad, but his girlfriend really drives me crazy. She constantly bugs me about all the things I should do differently. She lets up if Dad is around, but if he isn't, then it's pure torture! I eat constantly when I'm there because I figure if I keep my mouth full all the time, then maybe I won't say something I'll regret!

Our examples could go on and on, and you can undoubtedly come up with some of your own. The Stop, Drop and Roll tool can be very helpful during such times (see chapter 8). Examine situations in which you and your child repeatedly overeat, and consider whether habits or traditions may be playing a role. Talk openly about how you are affected by the emotions that are stirred within you, and then work together to develop family strategies so that you can avoid repeating the same mistakes over and over again. You might pray together before a family reunion, asking God to bless the family time and help you to obey your natural hunger and satisfaction signals. You and your child could develop a secret signal to use when either of you recognizes old habits taking over.

If your child has to deal with a difficult situation on her own, as Melissa did, then you might designate specific times that you will be praying for her. This will allow her to feel your love and the presence of God during those times when she is alone.

While prayer is always helpful in any situation, sometimes, as Dave and Ann recognized, drastic practical measures may be necessary as well.

We used to enjoy traveling to college football games nearly every weekend. We had a great time tailgating; spending time with friends and family; enjoying barbecued ribs, burgers, hot dogs, chips and desserts galore! But there were some obvious draw-backs—we ate the entire weekend, rarely exercised and often returned home exhausted. We tried to improve our eating choices, but each time we found ourselves falling into the same habits. After a time of prayer, we felt God was leading us to give up the football weekends. At first, it seemed like a rad-ical change, but we've been thrilled with the results! By stay-ing at home, we spend far less money, are able to enjoy relaxed activities, catch up on weekend chores and make much better food choices.

As you examine particular situations in your family's life, ask for God's discernment in understanding how to approach these circum-stances with greater wisdom. God will always make a way for you as you look to Him for guidance. "No temptation has overtaken you except such as is common to man; but God is faithful, who will not allow you to be tempted beyond what you are able, but with the temp-tation will also make the way of escape, that you may be able to bear it" (1 Cor. 10:13, *NKJV*).

Vacation and Holidays

Few things can destroy your good intentions like a vacation, a trip to the beach or a day at your favorite amusement park! Eating in restaurants three meals a day, especially if combined with an "I deserve it" attitude, is an automatic set-up for a big fall. Who wants to be the "Bad Mom" or the "Mean Dad" on vacation, reminding the kids to avoid second helpings and eat more fruits and vegetables? Unfortunately, one or two weeks of overindulgence can have long-lasting results.

Holidays represent a unique obstacle, because they blend together the relaxation of a vacation with the deeply ingrained traditions that we discussed earlier. Family get-togethers, parties, holiday baking, shopping and school functions all conspire to make exercise and appropriate eating *seem* impossible. Trying to cram in too many activities can easily lead us away from enjoying Whole-Body Pleasers, choosing instead those convenient—but unsatisfying—Taste-Bud Teasers. As a result, many of us just give up and accept a 10-pound weight gain as a normal part of the Christmas tradition!

While an important key to surviving leisure time is to keep "0 to 5" eating firmly in mind, you should also utilize the many other helpful tools now at your disposal. But a note to the wise: Your healthy eating tools will be much more effective if you examine your trouble spots ahead of time and have a workable strategy.

The Wilson family shares some positive changes they made to ensure healthy eating on their road trips.

When we hit the road in the past, we would immediately begin discussing where we would stop to eat. Now, we pack a picnic lunch, including beneficial food choices and beverages. When everyone is hungry, we stop at a rest area or a park (rather than a fast-food place) and enjoy a picnic. Afterward, we throw a Frisbee or toss a football. If the children become restless, we stop at a convenience market and let them buy a game or activity for the car. This allows us to stretch our legs, and gives the kids a treat, but leaves food out of the equation.

Tony bakes wonderful, "melt in your mouth" cookies every Christmas for friends and family. He truly enjoys it, and those who receive his cookies are deeply appreciative. Unfortunately, this baking tradition used to have a negative impact on his health and the health of his entire family because everyone would enjoy his cookies several times throughout the day—for weeks on end!

Tony's solution to the problem was simple: When the freshly baked cookies have cooled, they are immediately placed into a tin or gift bag for the recipient. A *few* cookies are set aside for the family, and any remaining cookies are placed directly into the freezer. This has allowed Tony to continue his gift-giving tradition, without compromising his health or that of his family.

As you approach the wonderful times of family vacations or holidays, ask God to help you prepare. Discuss problem areas with the entire family, including your kids. Children have amazing insight, but we often forget to seek their opinion. Write down ideas, and consider setting goals and rewards for each member of the family. Remember, if you are able to forego a fast-food meal while traveling and replace it with Whole-Body Pleasers and exercise, everyone deserves congratulations!

The Lurking Saboteurs

Many obstacles are predictable and easy to identify, but some of the biggest threats to our success are sneaky and subtle. A saboteur is "someone who commits sabotage or deliberately causes wrecks; a person who destroys, or ruins, or lays waste to." Synonyms include "ruiner," "uprooter" and "undoer."[2]

Are there any "ruiners" within your circle of family or friends? Nearly every family has one. A saboteur might be a person who feels threatened by change and wants to keep things just the way they are. A friendlier saboteur might be someone who unintentionally knocks you off the path toward fitness without any harmful intent.

Let's first consider people in your life who may be saboteurs. Does your child have a friend who deliberately encourages him to overeat? Is there a relative who is offended if you don't eat according to his or her expectations? ("But I baked this cake just for *you!*") If so, you are being subjected to sabotage. Only you can determine whether this issue can be directly addressed with the saboteur—many times it cannot or should not. However, it is vitally important that you develop a strategy for dealing with such sabotage.

If the sabotage is directed at your child, sit down and talk it over with her. She needs to recognize that her healthy eating habits are under attack. We recommend being kind to the other person, yet direct. Consider Susan's story.

At age 12, Susan enjoys being at her natural, God-ordained size. Although she was overweight as a young child, her family was introduced to the concepts of hunger and fullness several years ago, so now she eats only when she is hungry and stops when she is satisfied. This is easy at school because the food really isn't very good, so she looks forward to eating dinner at home with her family. Susan does not have an eating disorder and, in fact, is now a naturally thin person. However, as Susan relates, one of her friends—who is overweight—doesn't see it that way:

> I get so sick of hearing Misty tell me I need to eat more! She is constantly bugging me about it, trying to get me to eat every-thing on my plate. I try to tell her I'm not that hungry, but she just won't listen. The other day, she even accused me of being anorexic . . . right in front of all my friends!

What Susan is experiencing is an attempt by Misty to sabotage her. Ideally Misty would benefit from *following* Susan's eating habits rather than criticizing her—but with a saboteur, things often get turned upside down! Susan and her mom had a long talk about Misty's behavior, and together they devised some strategies for her to use while at school. Susan now avoids sitting next to Misty during lunch, if possible. But when she can't avoid it, she politely informs Misty that her parents and her doctor confirm that her weight is just right. She explains that she doesn't always like school food, so she sometimes eats just enough to get through the day and then enjoys a delicious dinner at home.

Prayer is an extremely important part of dealing with someone who is attempting to sabotage your efforts to raise a fit kid. Ask for God's guidance to understand the other person's motives. Consider whether your own behavior (or your child's) could be a part of the problem. Lastly, spend time praying for the person who is acting as the saboteur. Ask God to allow you to see this person from His perspective, to stand strong on the truth He has revealed to you and to show you ways to demonstrate His love toward this individual. At times, however, you might have to consider distancing yourself—or your child—from this person.

Another important saboteur isn't a person at all. It could be the television or other forms of media advertisement. In our high-tech world, television has become such a part of our daily lives that the furniture in most of our rooms is centered around it! And yet it is incredibly important to recognize the harmful effects that TV can have on your child. With proper supervision it can be enjoyable and harmless, but rest assured that failing to monitor your child's TV time will have a negative impact on his health.

Television influences children in many negative ways. It promotes an inactive lifestyle, as your child "lives out" adventure without ever lifting a finger. There are innumerable advertisements for food—nearly always Taste-Bud Teasers—and each can have a definite impact on your child's hunger level and on his ability to make wise food choices. In fact, studies indicate that the amount of television a child views each day has a direct impact on his weight gain, with each additional hour of TV viewing contributing to additional weight gain.[3] Lastly, much of the programming and advertisements on television promote the "I want it all" lifestyle that is so prevalent in our culture today.

For all of these reasons, we recommend that you take a long, hard look at your family's television viewing time. If the TV is clicked on within minutes of your entering the house, then it's likely your children are learning from you that silence is uncomfortable. Make gradual, consistent efforts to have more time together without the intrusion of technology (this means television, video games or computers). Eventually, you will spend more time conversing with each other, and perhaps even more time enjoying the outdoors together.

Other saboteurs include office "goodies," business lunches, class-room parties, all-you-can-eat buffets, potluck dinners, ice-cream socials, doughnuts after church and the kindly neighbor who just wants to share her homemade cookies every week. Whoever or what-ever the ruiner, you and your child can avoid getting tripped up if you recognize the sabotage and develop a strategy to undo the undoer.

Navigating Difficult Circumstances

The situations we have discussed are common obstacles that occur in nearly everyone's life at one time or another. However, some situations are far more complicated. Have you ever found yourself in a circum-stance that you never, ever thought would happen to you? Perhaps you have suffered through the pain of divorce and now face the challenge of raising a child alone. Maybe your family has experienced the tragedy of a serious illness or death from which you are still reeling. Or perhaps you have been caught in a severe financial crisis. Maybe a close family member is addicted to alcohol or drugs, and the entire family is on a roller coaster of frustration and fear.

If you are dealing with a serious challenge, you are probably already aware that children in these situations may feel their security threat-ened and respond in self-destructive ways. As their needs intensify, ten-sion and conflict may escalate, further threatening family stability.

Such extreme circumstances can make parents and children feel isolated and alone. Yet the fashionably dressed person sitting next to you in church that appears to have it all together may well be struggling with similar issues. So, if you are feeling alone, we encourage you to prayerfully consider in whom you might confide—perhaps a Christian friend or a pastor. Or you might decide to seek godly counsel through another avenue. Regardless of where you turn, we recommend that you take the first step toward breaking the painful cycle of isolation.

Second, consider how your difficult circumstances may be affect-ing your children. When serious trouble persists, children have a ten-dency to "hide" to avoid getting caught in the crossfire. As a result, your child's struggles may be overlooked, and you may find yourself unable to provide the stability and security that she requires. If this is the case, she may begin to look elsewhere to find the fulfillment and security that she needs. Sudden weight gain, uncontrolled spending, hanging out with shady friends or a change in personality can all be signs of a child in desperate need of time and attention. If any of these signs strikes a familiar chord with you, we encourage you to take it seriously and seek help for your family and your child.

We cannot pretend to have easy solutions or to truly understand your pain. However, there is One who knows your every struggle and feels your sadness as though it were His own. If a serious situation has rocked you to the core, leaving a hole in your heart, allow God to fill it as only He can. He promises that nothing can separate us from His love. Grab hold of that promise, hang on to it for dear life, and He will direct your path.

Plan of Action

We have discussed a number of challenges that life can throw our way. A basic plan of action can help you navigate the storms of life, regardless of the exact form they take.

Plan

As you recognize situations that threaten the Fit Kid lifestyle that you desire for your child, write each of these down. Then briefly review the tools that we have introduced throughout the book: the Tummy Keys, Belly Meter, Whole-Body Pleasers, Fun Jar, Motion Monitor, Word Wand, and Stop, Drop and Roll. Identify specific ways these tools can be utilized to help you prepare for the expected tough times of life. Make this a family activity so that kids can share in the planning as well as in the success. Set goals and establish rewards so that you can celebrate together when you successfully clear a hurdle that has tripped you up in the past.

Persevere

There are days when nothing seems to be working, regardless of all our best efforts. In those times, our best strategy is to simply keep going. Our response to life isn't always pretty, but the willingness to hang in there and stay the course pays off in the long run. It is *always* darkest just before dawn. When you feel you simply cannot take another step forward, your breakthrough may be just around the corner.

Pray

Whether your obstacle is just a bump in the road or what appears to be an insurmountable mountain, commit your struggle to God through prayer. Take your issues to God's throne and have a heart-to-heart, pouring out your fears and worries to Him. Not only will He listen, but He will also give you the specific answers you need. God has promised that He will never forsake us during times of trouble, will never allow us to be tempted beyond what we are able to endure, will always provide for us a means of escape, and will direct our paths when we seek His will. God's response to dedicated prayer promises to be more than you can imagine or hope for.

Eternal Perspective

In hindsight, we can often recognize suffering as a blessing, a time when we drew closer to God and our loved ones, and learned the life lessons that truly matter. An unknown Confederate soldier said to have been seriously disabled during the Civil War expressed his feelings about hardship this way:

> I asked God for strength, that I might achieve,
> I was made weak, that I might learn humbly to obey.
> I asked for health, that I might do greater things,
> I was given infirmity that I might do better things.
> I asked for riches, that I might be happy,
> I was given poverty, that I might be wise.
> I asked for power, that I might have the praise of men,
> I was given weakness, that I might feel the need of God.
> I asked for all things, that I might enjoy life,
> I was given life, that I might enjoy all things.
> I got nothing that I asked for—but everything I had hoped for.
> Almost despite myself, my unspoken prayers were answered.
> I am, among all men, most richly blessed.[4]

As you face whatever lies ahead, we pray that you will see your circumstances with the eyes of faith, trusting that God will walk with you always and carry you when necessary.

Lord, we come to You asking for guidance
as we struggle through the challenges that come our way.
Please direct us toward the narrow path that leads to You.
Help us to avoid following the crowd of people
who seek only to please themselves.
Strengthen us as we falter, and help us to trust that
there is nothing too hard for You.
Amen.

I have told you all this so that you may
have peace in me. Here on earth you will have many
trials and sorrows. But take heart,
because I have overcome the world.

JOHN 16:33

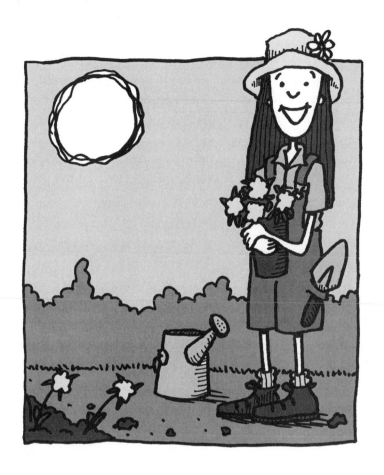

CHAPTER 11

KICK IT UP A NOTCH

Expanding the Fit Kid Principles to Other Areas

What in the world does '0 to 5' eating have to do with how I spend my money?" Kai asked his mom. Kelsey's 15-year-old son, Kai, was the perfect example of a naturally thin person who enjoys food but eats only according to his body's cues for hunger and satisfaction. However, his spending habits were an *entirely* different matter. Regardless of his parents' efforts to help him save money, Kai spent every dime he earned—usually on frivolous things. He wouldn't save a cent unless his parents put it in a savings account for him.

But Kelsey finally made a connection between Kai's spending and his eating habits. She pointed out to Kai how he respects and honors his body by choosing beneficial foods in the right amounts and by being physically active. They discussed how he rarely eats Taste-Bud Teasers because he prefers Whole-Body Pleasers.

Then Kelsey compared these wise eating habits to his spending habits, describing how he frequently spends money on "teasers" (or even Total Rejects) so that he never has money for the quality items he desires. Kelsey suggested that Kai practice self-restraint in the area of money management—the same self-restraint that had been so effective when it came to eating. Amazingly enough, the conversation seemed to make an impact, and Kai began to make great progress toward spending wisely.

Giving our kids a concept or picture that they can easily grasp—as Kelsey did for her son—can be a lifesaver when it comes to teaching children these valuable lessons. Let's look at how the principles learned in earlier chapters can become teaching points in other areas of life, such as financial responsibility, developing a heart for service and making wise career choices.

Raising a Financially Fit Kid

Learning to handle money responsibly is an extremely important lesson for our children. Kids growing up in our culture are bombarded with all sorts of messages about how to spend their money—and only rarely on how to save, invest or give.

Temptations and obstacles that lure us to overeat can also lure us to overspend. Living in a society with a superabundance of wealth and a poor understanding of how to be good stewards of money puts young people at risk of making potentially serious mistakes. If we don't want our grown children up to their eyeballs in debt by the time they are 25, then it is necessary to train them to handle finances in a godly way while they are still young. And it is never too early to begin.

Consider the story of Steve and Renee:

> We were both raised in Christian homes, but we didn't receive a lot of instruction from our parents about money management. When we married, we felt as if we deserved nice things, like so many other couples we knew. We borrowed as much as we could in order to purchase our first home and then used credit cards to furnish it. Even though we both had student loans to repay, we frequently ate out at restaurants and also bought a new car. Before we knew it, we were drowning in debt, even though both of us had good jobs. Now we really want to have children, but we honestly don't think we can afford to do so.

None of us wants to see our children end up in Steve and Renee's position, with the American Dream turned into a nightmare of debt. Had Steve and Renee been appropriately prepared at home or had some financial counseling, many of their mistakes could have been avoided. There are wonderful resources available to teach children how to handle money appropriately, and some of the Fit Kids principles we have already applied to eating can be directed to finances as well.

1. It All Belongs to God

First and foremost we must recognize that everything we have belongs to God. The Bible tells us that everything—our bodies, worldly possessions, gifts and our success—all come from God and belong to God. Consider these words from the Old Testament and then seek to communicate these truths to your children as they apply to finances and material possessions:

> Lord, you are great and powerful. You have glory, victory, and honor. Everything in heaven and on earth belongs to you.

The kingdom belongs to you, Lord; you are the ruler over everything. Riches and honor come from you. You rule everything. You have the power and strength to make anyone great and strong (1 Chron. 29:11-12, NCV).

We live in a culture that has been blessed with wealth and success, yet we all know someone who was living the high life one moment, only to lose it all the next. As we faithfully provide for our children, let's take every opportunity to help them understand that the true source of all our provisions is God alone.

2. Heed Hunger and Satisfaction

As a family, develop the habit of asking a very simple question each time you make a purchase: "Is this something I *need*, or something I *want*?" As we have discussed previously, our actions speak far louder than our words! During this journey together, we hope that your child is learning to wait for true hunger before eating. In the same manner, he can apply the hunger principle to his purchases, asking himself if his desire to buy something is based on a genuine need ("Am I truly hungry?")—or because it's the latest fad and his friends all have that item ("Do I want to eat even though I'm not really hungry?"). The patience to wait for God to meet our needs is essential as we seek to practice financial responsibility.

Sally is an eighth-grade student whose parents are divorced. She is known among her friends as the "cell-phone queen" because every time a new model comes out, her father buys it for her—she has nine so far! Because she travels between her parents' separate households, the first mobile phone may have been appropriate. However, being provided the "better, faster, quicker" models reinforces the idea that she must *always* have the latest and greatest. Not only does this foster a lack of contentment, but it also creates an expectation that will be difficult to meet in the long run.

Eating when one isn't hungry overrides the reliable system God set up to tell us how much is adequate nourishment for our bodies. Likewise, purchasing the latest model gadget "just because it's there" overrides a person's sense of what is really needed and feeds greed. It is difficult for our children to say, "I am satisfied!" when they are consistently provided with a faster, better, flashier model of this or that. Consider where it will end if we don't teach our children to exercise self-control and to feed *need* instead of *want*.

3. Make Wise Choices

Every single purchase you make, large or small, can be used to help your child understand how to make wise financial choices. A new toy that quickly falls apart demonstrates the importance of quality over flashy appearances (of course, this lesson may need to wait until after the tears dry!). Reviewing the mortgage bill with older children helps them understand the importance of long-term investments. And sharing with our kids the difference between paying cash verses credit for a new TV allows them to appreciate the *real* cost of using credit cards for instant gratification.

As is true with all of us, the most effective lessons will be those that your child learns when spending her *own* money! When four-year-old Gracie wanted a stuffed animal that she saw in the store, she faithfully saved her money until the day finally arrived when she could buy the toy. She walked into the store, happily picked out the long-awaited prize, marched to the counter and proudly handed the clerk her money. But when the clerk placed the toy in a bag and gave it to her, Gracie stood at the counter for a moment with an uncertain expression on her face, then tearfully turned to her mother and cried out, "Mommy, he *kept* my money!" It was her first real experience with making a purchase on her own, and she simply didn't understand that she wouldn't be getting her money back. Ever since that day, Gracie and her money have not been easily parted!

As your child learns to evaluate how much he wants something, he will begin to develop more patience. Be sure to affirm him when you see him set aside instant gratification in favor of a wiser choice for the future.

4. Evaluate Heart Hunger

In the daily hustle and bustle of school projects, baseball games and homework, it is easy for us to overlook the inner longings of our child's hearts. If you notice your child suddenly splurging on inconsequential things, this might be a red flag that she has an emotional ache in her heart.

Likewise, it is important for parents to avoid using money to try to meet the deeper needs that our children have. In the example of "the cell-phone queen," Sally's father may have bought her the newest and coolest cell phones in order to make up for not spending enough time with her. The sad truth is that Sally probably desires a more intimate relationship with her dad, not another new cell phone.

In his letter to the Philippians, Paul describes living at both ends of the spectrum of hunger and satisfaction, and he gives us a wonderful glimpse of how life can be lived when we turn to Christ for our ultimate needs, rather than trying to satisfy our heart hunger with money or possessions.

> I have learned to be satisfied with the things I have and with everything that happens. I know how to live when I am poor, and I know how to live when I have plenty. I have learned the secret of being happy at any time in everything that happens, when I have enough to eat and when I go hungry, when I have more than I need and when I do not have enough. I can do all things through Christ, because he gives me strength (Phil. 4:11-13, *NCV*).

May we strive in our own lives—and may we teach our children—to lay hold of this truth: A God-centered life frees us from the bondage of worldly living and allows us to embark on an adventure filled with contentment, excitement and passion.

Bringing It Home

Some families teach their children from an early age how to calculate 10 percent of any dollar earned and to set this amount aside for God. This allows children to bring their first fruits to God, learning not to hold on too tightly to that which has been so freely given. Helping children understand the ways that their donations are put to use can then help them to gain an understanding of God's community at work.

The Andersons tell this story:

When the kids were only four and six years old, the church that we attended began a campaign to build a new children's center. Leah and Jonathan eagerly did extra chores for us and our neighbors, filling their piggy bank to contribute to the building fund. Even though that was eight years ago and we've since moved, whenever we pass our old church, the kids comment about how they helped to build that beautiful center for all the children that now enjoy it! They have a sense of having been a part of something bigger than themselves.

Helping our children to see *others* and *eternity*, rather than *me* and *now* is an invaluable gift that will lead them to greater financial responsibility and contentment.

Raising a Child with a Heart for Service

In chapter 7, we explained the importance of an active lifestyle in achieving fitness. It's tough to raise a fit kid while sitting on the couch! In the same way, when we exercise faith and put it into action, we demonstrate a spiritually active lifestyle for our children. When given a good example, children can learn to put their faith into action, as Jesus described when He said, "You will be my witnesses in Jerusalem, and in all Judea and Samaria, and to the ends of the earth" (Acts 1:8, *NIV*).

Beginning locally, right in your own neighborhood or church—your "Jerusalem"—you can show your kids how to consider the needs of others. You might volunteer to fold bulletins at the church, help serve at a special event, do roadside cleanup or take meals to those in need through Meals on Wheels. You might not have to look beyond your next-door neighbor to find someone in need that you and your child can serve or encourage.

One family's car time allowed them to become more spiritually active:

When our children were seven and nine, my husband and I wanted them to see firsthand that people don't always have a nice home, two cars and a dog. They had known nothing of poverty or homelessness, so we drove through a part of town where there was a rescue mission and long lines for hot meals. Our children were surprised to realize that there were so many people without even enough money to buy a meal for themselves. This definitely opened our children's eyes and set the stage for our family to volunteer together at the rescue mission and at a homeless women's shelter.

Another family heard of the terrible devastation in a nearby town that had been hit by a hurricane. They participated in a massive community collection effort, and their 12- and 14-year-old boys were able to make the 3-hour journey to deliver food and clothing to those in need. It was an experience these young men would not soon forget, as they reached out to their "Judea and Samaria."

Three families, including kids ranging from 5 to 19 years of age, loaded up their vans and trucks and headed to an orphanage in Mexico for a week during the summer. While there, they ministered to the needs of the children and staff at the orphanage, in effect reaching "to the ends of the earth."

As kids have opportunities to serve others, they will begin to discover their passions, gifts, talents and skills. They will see that God has made them in a unique way for a distinct purpose. One young lady had no idea she had a knack for storytelling until she helped out in the kindergarten Sunday School class at church. The children remained riveted during story time, as this 12-year-old girl presented Bible stories with animation and gusto! God said that there are things that He has prepared in advance for each of us to do (see Eph. 2:10). As we guide our children into a broad range of experiences to serve God and others, they will see situations as opportunities for growth and ministry, and will begin to develop mature and tender hearts of mercy.

Bringing It Home
As a family, consider contributing time or resources to well-respected organizations: Angel Tree, Samaritan's Purse, Meals on Wheels, or some

other well-known, well-organized cause. Sponsoring a child through an organization of your choice doesn't require much time or money—and can make a big difference in another's life. Setting aside one day a month to serve meals at a homeless shelter is doable for most families and is an experience your kids won't soon forget. The bottom line here: *Exercise your faith by putting it into action—reach out to those who are in need!*

Can you think of someone with a specific need that your family can meet? Or is there a service project, church work or community service that you and your kids might get involved with, even for an hour this month? Write some ideas in the space below.

_____

_____

_____

_____

_____

_____

_____

_____

_____

_____

_____

_____

Preparing for a Career

While we may not know the best way to encourage our children to consider their future, thankfully God does—and He has something perfect in mind: " 'For I know the plans I have for you,' says the LORD. 'They are plans for good and not for disaster, to give you a future and a hope'" (Jer. 29:11).

As parents, it is our job to provide our children with as many opportunities as possible for nurturing their talents and spiritual gifts. This will provide them with a resource from which to draw as God directs them further down the road of life. Of course, if we are honest, being open to allowing our kids to discern their own path is not without challenges for many of us. Truthfully, our interests are often somewhat conflicted. Sometimes as parents we genuinely enjoy our careers—and we just want our children to share our passion and follow in our footsteps. Unfortunately, we don't always stop to consider the heartfelt desires of our kids.

Jim vividly recalls that when he was growing up, he wanted to be an elementary school teacher. But his physician father absolutely loved his career and wanted Jim to be a doctor, hoping they would eventually practice medicine together. Jim says, "I loved and respected my father, but I didn't share his passion for medicine. However, I reluctantly did what he wanted and became a doctor. Unfortunately, Dad died before we were ever able to practice together. Now I feel trapped in my career, but my dream to be an elementary school teacher still calls out to me."

Everyone would agree that Jim is successful. Yet frequently he wonders whether he experiences God's best for his life because he chose a profession with an eye toward pleasing his earthly father rather than his heavenly Father.

On the other hand, if we want our children to avoid mistakes we've made, we may push them in the opposite direction. Our attempts to run interference may then stand in the way of the realization of God's plan for our children.

In still other cases, we might see our children's decisions as a reflection of our parenting skills. We may desire that their choices bring us accolades and praise, without regard for whether those choices reflect God's will for their lives.

In an effort to avoid these pitfalls, let's apply some of the Fit Kid principles to this area of our lives.

1. Ask the Right Question

Even at a very young age, children are frequently asked, "What do you want to be when you grow up?" Perhaps we're asking the wrong question. As we accept the sacred honor of raising "fit" children to become what God intends them to be, the better question may be, *What is God's purpose for your life?*

God created your child with unique gifts, desires and abilities, and He has a specific purpose in mind for your child. As you and your child consider the future, ask God's guidance for understanding how these qualities can best be developed. Ask Him how you can provide opportunities for your child's innate gifts to be fanned into flame or new skills to be discovered and developed that will help him to know his calling later in life.

2. Choose Whole-Body Pleasers
One really cool thing about kids is that they place absolutely no limits on their aspirations (or lack thereof!). Children may pick a career at age four and never look back, while other children's lack of focus may cause their parents to worry that they are raising a professional video-game player! Consider some of the career aspirations of a few recent preschool graduates:

- A sea captain, a nurse *and* a doctor —Jessica, age 5
- A "ringer upper" at a Target store —Kendal, age 4
- A mommy —Sarah, age 4
- A princess —Kendall, age 5
- A boxer —Griffin, age 5
- A veterinarian —Gracie, age 6
- A cowboy —James, age 5

Of course, at this age these kids might also have listed gummy bears, chicken nuggets and chocolate chip cookies as their favorite foods! An important task as we navigate the roller coaster of parenting will be to help our children develop an awareness of the unlimited possibilities available to them.

In chapter 6, we discussed the concept of Whole-Body Pleasers, which are foods that taste terrific, are satisfying and offer wholesome goodness for the body. This is a helpful concept to keep in mind as you and your child discuss her future. Some careers might be more like Taste-Bud Teasers, offering instant gratification and a big burst of POW!, but not be particularly satisfying in the long run or beneficial in providing all the things she needs. Other careers might be very useful and worthwhile, but the idea of spending a lifetime doing that job might turn your child's stomach.

We want children to gravitate toward a future that will be a Whole-Body Pleaser *for them*. As with foods, everyone's Whole-Body Pleaser career may be different. Yet we can rest assured that God will not call our children to do something they are incapable of doing.

From an early age, Shana wanted to be a professional singer. She read and came to know many personal details about singing stars in every musical genre, from classical to country. As she got older, one problem arose: She really couldn't sing. In fact, she sounded like one of those early auditions for *American Idol*. This deficiency was not something that could be remedied with formal voice training. Eventually Shana resigned herself to singing for pleasure and decided she would have to look for a career elsewhere. For Shana, singing was a career that "tasted great," but God clearly had other plans for her—she simply didn't have the gifts and abilities necessary to pull off a singing career.

3. Eat Lots of Fruit

"The Spirit produces the fruit of love, joy, peace, patience, kindness, goodness, faithfulness, gentleness, self-control" (Gal. 5:22, *NCV*). Throughout our time together, we have discussed character traits to encourage you to become the parent God desires you to be. Now it's time to consider how to foster the development of these character traits in your children.

Children who develop these deeper attributes at an early age have a firm foundation on which to build their adult lives. Patience and self-control (not commonly observed in our society) are extremely beneficial character qualities, especially when kids are faced with studying difficult school subjects or learning a complex profession. Practicing kindness and goodness teaches your child to reach out to others and to experience the true joy of service. The more these spiritual attributes are developed, the more likely your child is to choose a future that is in line with God's plan for his life.

As you encourage the growth and maturity of spiritual fruit in your child, she will respond best by observing your actions. It will be difficult for your daughter to produce "Golden Delicious apples" if she sees only "sour grapes" at home! On the other hand, if *you* are growing closer to God, studying the Bible and sharing God's Word with your children, there is a good probability that she will become a miniature fruit tree, bearing her own delicious fruit in the likeness of our Lord.

Bringing It Home
Expose your children to a variety of professions, vocations or trades. Allow them to spend time with professionals from different fields and to ask questions that truly interest them. Provide exposure to new ideas (within reason, of course), as well as volunteer opportunities. One 12-year-old who volunteered to be a "junior curator" at a local science museum grew up to be a full-fledged curator! She may have never developed an interest without that priceless childhood experience.

Let Go and Let God

One of the most difficult aspects of parenting is allowing children to make their own decisions. While a toddler requires your constant supervision and hands-on care, your teenagers may feel suffocated with the same amount of attention. The level of help your child needs to make decisions regarding a career, relationships or finances depends on his age and maturity. Your task as a parent is to prepare the soil, to build a solid foundation on God's Word and to provide your child with structure, discipline and godly guidance.

When children are very young, it is easy for us to believe that we can form them into whatever shape we choose. They seem so dependent on our opinions and so responsive to our guidance. Even when they disobey us, it remains clear that what we think about them *really matters*. But as our children grow and mature, our influence diminishes daily, like sand slipping through our fingers, and the influence of the world increases.

Many of us can relate to Diane's story about her son Kevin:

I just could not believe how everything changed when Kevin began kindergarten! Until then, I was his favorite person on the earth . . . he wouldn't choose an ice-cream flavor or an outfit without my approval! Suddenly the opinions that mattered

most to him were those of his teacher and his friends. It isn't
that I wanted him to stay a baby forever, but I just wasn't prepared for how quickly things would change!

As we point our children toward the God of the universe, we can
pray for their growth and trust that being rooted in God's Word and
ways will help them make good choices regarding lifestyle, finances,
careers and relationships. We can pray, too, that we will respect their
decisions, entrusting their care and protection to the sovereign hands
of a loving Lord.

Lord, You have placed these precious children under our protection,
and it is such an awesome task! May we prepare them well,
and may we guide them down the path of Your choosing.
Please grant us Your peace as we allow them to make important choices.
We entrust them to You and place them into Your loving hands.
Amen.

God's love, though, is ever and always,
eternally present to all who fear him,
making everything right for them and their
children as they follow his covenant ways and
remember to do whatever he said.

PSALM 103:17-18, *THE MESSAGE*

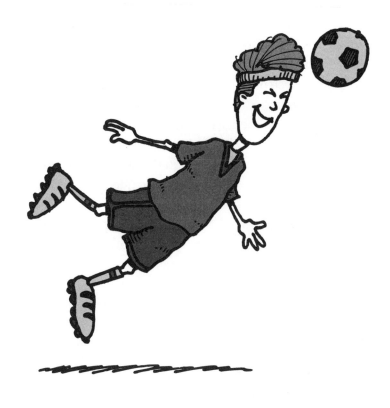

CHAPTER 12

A TIME TO SOAR

Where You Have Come from and
Where You Are Going

I n our time together, we have covered a *lot* of territory. We have pondered the amusing antics of children, the frustrating confusion of parenting, and heartbreaking issues such as death and divorce. We've considered hunger and fullness, carbohydrates and cholesterol, activity and exercise. We've traveled from the ball field to holiday parties, through Disneyland vacations, right into the home of stepparents. We have reflected on *life*—the good times, the bad times and all those in-between times. You now have the tools needed to raise a *whole child*—one who is fit on the outside and fulfilled on the inside.

Your real journey has only just begun, and this is an opportunity for you to recognize and rejoice in the progress you and your child have made. In order to do this, we have included some of the questionnaire from chapter 2. As you complete these questions, it is our heartfelt prayer that you will see and celebrate important changes that have taken place in your family's eating and exercise habits, methods of communication, and your spiritual journey.

Please answer the following questions using a scale of 0 to 10, with "0" meaning "never" and "10" meaning "always."

Can you visualize your child as trim or healthy? _____
Is food and/or your child's weight a source of conflict? _____
Do you frequently check your child's weight? _____
Do you allow your child to eat whatever and whenever he wants? _____

For the questions below, please circle the answer that best describes your situation.

When eating, are you aware of *your* body's hunger and fullness signals?
Yes, Always   Sort of   **No way—my body has those?**

Does *your child* seem to realize when he is hungry, satisfied and full?
Definitely   Maybe   **You're kidding, right?**

Do *you* wait for true hunger before eating?
Always   **Usually**   **Sometimes**   **Never**

Does *your child* wait for true hunger before eating?
Always   Usually   Sometimes   Never

Do *you* stop eating when satisfied, before becoming too full?
Always   Usually   Sometimes   Never

Does *your child* stop eating when satisfied, before becoming too full?
Always   Usually   Sometimes   Never

Do *you* normally finish everything on your plate?
Never   Sometimes   Often   Always

Does *your child* usually finish everything on her plate?
Absolutely Not   Sometimes   Often   Always

Does your child have to eat all of his food to get dessert?
Never   Sometimes   Often   Always

Do you and your child have power struggles over food choices?
Never   Occasionally   Often   At every meal

Next, imagine your stomach as a balloon and answer the following questions using a scale of 0 to 10. A "0" is when the balloon is completely empty, while a "10" is when the balloon is completely filled up to the point it is about to pop.

I normally *start* eating at a _____.
I normally *stop* eating at a _____.
My child usually *starts* eating at a _____.
My child usually *stops* eating at a _____.

Answer the following questions using a scale of 0 to 10. This time, "0" means "never" and "10" means "always."

Our family eats on the run. _____
Our family eats separately rather than together. _____

Our family eats somewhere *other than* the dinner table. _____

Our family eats fast food. _____

Our family eats out at restaurants. _____

Our meals involve arguments or conflict. _____

Our family celebrates with food. _____

Our family eats for emotional reasons. _____

Family outings are planned around food. _____

My child eats due to stress or boredom. _____

My child eats because of unhappiness or sadness. _____

My child overeats in social situations (with friends, at parties, at sporting events, and so on). _____

My child prefers eating alone. _____

My child eats in front of the TV or computer. _____

My own bad eating habits seem to affect my child. _____

In general, how do you rate your life in the following areas? Again, answer using a scale of 0 to 10. "0" means terrible and "10" means wonderful.	*In general, how do you rate your child's life in the following areas? Again, answer using a scale of 0 to 10. "0" means terrible and "10" means wonderful.*
Overall health _____	Overall health _____
Energy level _____	Energy level _____
Self-esteem _____	Self-esteem _____
Job satisfaction (consider student or homemaker as a job) _____	Success in school and/or work _____
Outside interests _____	Talents/success in extracurricular activities _____
Marriage/romantic relationships _____	Relationships with parents _____
Relationship with your children _____	Relationships with siblings _____
Close relationships/friendships _____	Close relationships/friendships _____
Communication skills _____	Communication skills _____
Overall happiness _____	Overall happiness _____
Relationship with God _____	Relationship with God _____

Compare your answers to those from the questionnaire in chapter 2. What positive changes can you celebrate? What additional adjustments would you still like to make?

God *is* doing a new thing, according to His Word (see Isa. 43:19). You and your child have taken the first steps toward health and wholeness, the benefits of which will continue for a lifetime. We rejoice and celebrate your successes with you!

Now let's look at what we call the Fat World Triangle to clarify what you have chosen to leave behind.

FAT WORLD TRIANGLE

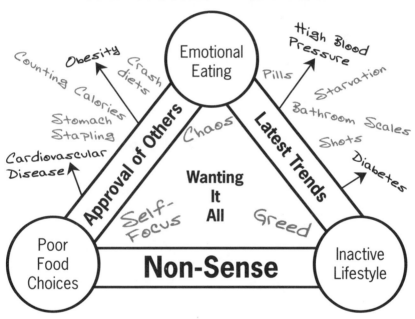

This triangle is built and supported by the *"non*sense" that the world spews forth, attempting to convince us that we can have it all by striving for the appearance of success. The messages that come from TV, magazines and the Internet tempt us to follow the latest fads and to compare ourselves to others. These harmful messages beg us to grab for a quick fix so that we might have everything we want, exactly when we want it. Without loving guidance, our children are not immune to this seduction.

Eating for emotional reasons, basing food choices only on taste and convenience, and an inactive lifestyle lead to children and adults who are far from fit. Comparing ourselves to others and focusing on outward appearance can lead to radical dieting. Families desperately seeking change may try anything and everything the media offers: counting calories, liquid diets, gastric bypass surgery, and a host of other drastic measures. For years we have been sold this defective bill of goods, and the grim statistics tell the tale of those, including children, who are suffering the consequences. This is *not* what God intends for His beloved children. He desires us to break free from this kind of chaotic living—and He has provided the way of escape. As you apply the Fit Kids principles you have learned, your dear child now has the amazing opportunity to discover that God can work wonders in even the most challenging of circumstances.

As a review of all that we have shared with you in this book, let's compare what the world offers, the Fat World Triangle, with what God offers, the Fit Kids Triangle below.

FIT KIDS TRIANGLE

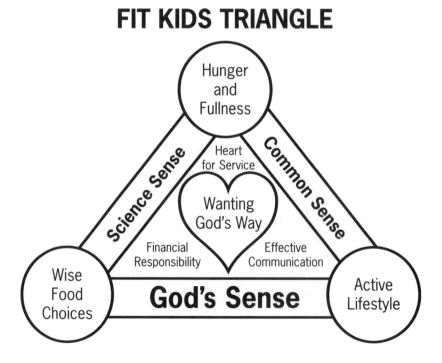

A life lived according to Fit Kid principles is built on a solid foundation of God's Word and on a living, breathing relationship with Him. We base our lives primarily on *God's* sense, supplemented by *common* sense and *science* sense. In doing so, we develop healthy, God-honoring habits that lead to balance and order in *all* areas of life. We embrace God's view of our bodies as "fearfully and wonderfully made," and we encourage our children to learn to recognize feelings of hunger and fullness so that they can eat the right amount of food. No longer lured only by what their taste buds dictate, children can choose and enjoy foods that taste terrific, are satisfying *and* offer wholesome nutrition to their bodies—Whole-Body Pleasers! We reject the sedentary lifestyle that is so prevalent and embrace an active life of discovery and adventure that will enrich our interaction with our children at all ages and stages.

Recognizing the deeper needs of our children, we seek to connect with them through our words and actions so that we might enjoy the deep, fulfilling relationship for which our hearts yearn. Aware now that unfulfilled "heart hunger" may draw us to food when we don't need it, we instead turn to God to meet our deeper needs.

Walking hand in hand with the Lord, and allowing Him to direct our paths, parents and children alike grow healthier physically, spiritually and emotionally. This is a lot to celebrate!

Carpe Diem! Seize the Day! *Go for It!*

Our deepest desire isn't to survive, but to thrive! We long to give life our all, knowing that we have enjoyed each day and lived it to the fullest. Erma Bombeck expressed this desire so well:

> I always had a dream that when I am asked to give an accounting of my life to a higher court, it will go like this: "So, empty your pockets. What have you got left of your life? Any dreams that were unfulfilled? Any unused talent that we gave you when you were born that you still have left? Any unsaid compliments or bits of love that you haven't spread around?" And I will answer, "I've nothing to return. I spent everything you gave me. I'm as naked as the day I was born."[1]

As parents, we don't want to look back on these precious years and remember the laundry or the long days at work. Instead, we long to savor each sacred moment with those precious gifts God has so graciously entrusted to us: our children.

God has *placed eternity in our hearts*. With this sentiment in mind, take life by storm and go for it with God as your guide! May you say, as does Eric Little in *Chariots of Fire*, "I run to feel God's pleasure!"[2] Press on as you continue to lead your child down the path of truth, pointing her toward the ultimate source of freedom so that she might sense God's pleasure and learn what it means to truly *live*!

As you contemplate the future for your family, may you and your child walk in God's will and live free from the captivity of a world driven toward outward perfection. May you know that through Him, *all things are indeed possible*. May you encourage your child to trust, to risk, to dance . . . *to soar*. For a child who knows God and understands truth, who is surrounded by love and who has the freedom to fly, the future is without limits.

> *O Father, as a deer pants for the water,*
> *may we hunger and thirst for You.*
> *May we raise our children in Your image,*
> *rather than in the image of the world.*
> *May they know You, the one true God,*
> *and Jesus Christ, whom You have sent.*
> *May they run without restraint, dance freely*
> *and soar with the wings of eagles.*
> *Amen.*

> The LORD says, "All you who are thirsty, come and drink.
> Those of you who do not have money, come, buy and eat!
> Come buy wine and milk without money and without cost.
> Why spend your money on something that is not real food?
> Why work for something that doesn't really satisfy you?
> Listen closely to me, and you will eat what is good;
> your soul will enjoy the rich food that satisfies.
> Come to me and listen; *listen to me so you may live*."
>
> ISAIAH 55:1-3, *NCV, EMPHASIS ADDED*

CALCULATING YOUR CHILD'S BODY MASS INDEX

CALCULATING YOUR CHILD'S BMI PERCENTILE

THE EIGHT TUMMY KEYS

VITAMINS

Calculating Your Child's Body Mass Index

If you are unable to obtain your child's BMI number from his doctor, it may be calculated several different ways. Regardless of which method you use, you will need a *current and accurate* reading of your child's height and weight, as even a slight variance (especially in height) can affect the BMI. If you use older measurements (such as from a prior checkup), make sure that you use your child's age *at that visit* (rather than current age) to obtain an accurate BMI.

1. *Online BMI Calculators.* Many websites provide a BMI calculator. You simply enter your child's age, sex, height and weight and you will then be provided the BMI. Some online calculators also provide the BMI percentile so that you won't need to use the charts below. An online BMI calculator can be found by typing "calculate body mass index" into any search engine, and the U.S. Center for Disease Control and Prevention (CDC) provides a calculator that can be found at http://apps.nccd.cdc.gov/dnpabmi/Calculator.aspx.

2. *BMI Charts.* The BMI may also be determined by referring to BMI charts, which indicate your child's BMI based on her height and weight. BMI charts for children ages 2 to 18 are available from the CDC at: http://www.cdc.gov/nccdphp/dnpa/bmi/00binaries/bmi-tables.pdf.

3. *Mathematic Calculation.* A third option is to calculate your child's BMI based on a mathematic formula, as follows:

   • Weight in pounds, divided by height in inches, divided *again* by height in inches = _____

   • Answer above multiplied by 703 = _____
     The result is your child's BMI.

As an example, let's assume David is 3 feet, 6 inches (42 inches) tall and weighs 43.5 pounds. To calculate his BMI, divide his weight in pounds (43.5) by his height in inches (42), and divide this *again* by his height in inches (42) = 0.0247. Next, multiply this number by 703 = *17.4*.

Calculating Your Child's BMI Percentile

Using your child's BMI number, you are now able to determine his BMI percentile using the charts developed by the CDC (see pages 224 and 225).[1] Find the correct chart for your child's sex (Figure 1 for boys and Figure 2 for girls); the correct age listed along the bottom of the chart; the correct BMI number listed along the left and right sides of the chart; and make a dot where those lines intersect. Next, follow the curved line out to the right to read your child's BMI percentile, ranging from third to ninety-seventh percentile.

Let's again use David as an example, whose BMI we calculated to be 17.4. When placed onto the boy's BMI percentile chart, David's BMI is just above the eighty-fifth percentile. So, what do these numbers mean? In David's case, this means that out of 100 boys who are four years old, David's BMI is higher than that of 85 boys and is lower than that of 15 boys.

According to CDC guidelines, a BMI at or above the ninety-fifth percentile is considered *obese;* a BMI from the eighty-fifth to ninety-fifth percentile is considered *overweight*; a BMI from the fifth to eighty-fifth percentile is considered at a *healthy weight*; and a BMI that is below the fifth percentile is considered *underweight*. Based on these categories, David's BMI percentile places him in the *overweight* category.

Based on the above, fill in your child's numbers:

My child's BMI is _____.
My child's BMI percentile is _____.
My child's BMI category is (circle one):

Obese   Overweight   Healthy weight   Underweight

Figure 1
CDC Growth Charts: United States

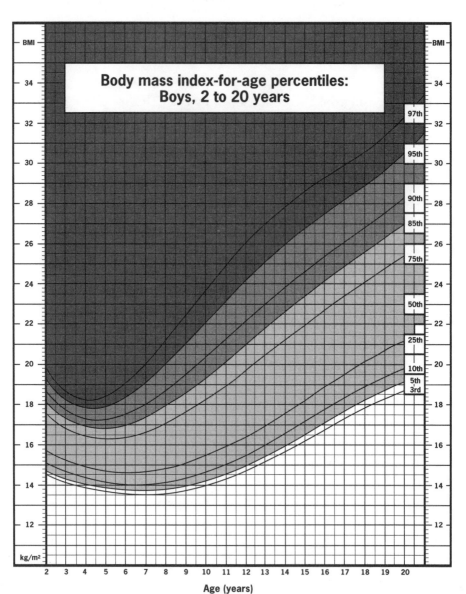

Figure 2
CDC Growth Charts: United States

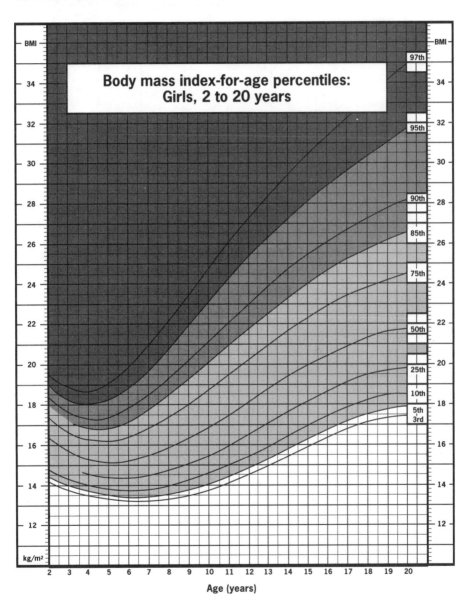

Body mass index-for-age percentiles:
Girls, 2 to 20 years

The Eight Tummy Keys

Use the charts below to help chart your progress with applying the Tummy Keys from chapter 3. Feel free to personalize the charts with decorations and stickers!

Tummy Keys	Mon	Tue	Wed	Thu	Fri	Sat	Sun
Key #1: My child waited for an empty tummy before eating.							
Key #2: My child sat down to eat.							
Key #3: We pressed the "mute button" while eating.							
Key #4: We remembered to pray together before eating.							
Key #5: We ate slowly and enjoyed each bite.							
Key #6: My child enjoyed yummy food.							
Key #7: My child demonstrated good manners.							
Key #8: My child stopped eating before feeling stuffed.							

Vitamins

Refer to the table below for additional information regarding common food sources of vitamins.[2]

Fat-Soluble Vitamins	
Vitamin A	Spinach and other green leafy vegetables
Cheese	Vegetable oils and products made from vegetable oils, such as margarine
Cod	Wheat germ
Cream	
Eggs	
Halibut fish oil	**Vitamin K**
Kidney	Cabbage
Liver	Cauliflower
Meat	Cereals
Milk	Soybeans
	Spinach
Vitamin D	**Water-Soluble Vitamins**
Butter	
Cereals	**Folate**
Cheese	Fortified foods
Cream	Green, leafy vegetables
Fish	
Fortified milk	**Niacin (B3)**
Margarine	Dairy products
Oysters	Eggs
	Enriched breads and cereals
Vitamin E	Fish
Asparagus	Lean meats
Corn	Legumes
Nuts	Nuts
Olives	Poultry
Seeds	

Pantothenic Acid and Biotin
Broccoli and other vegetables in the
    cabbage family
Dairy products
Eggs
Fish
Lean beef
Legumes
White and sweet potatoes
Whole-grain cereals
Yeast

Thiamine (B1)
Dairy products
Dried beans
Fish
Fortified breads, cereals and pasta
Fruits and vegetables
Lean meats
Peas
Soybeans
Whole grains

Vitamin B12
Eggs
Meat
Milk and milk products
Poultry
Shellfish

Vitamin C (ascorbic acid)
Broccoli
Cantaloupe
Citrus fruits and juices
Strawberries
Sweet and white potatoes
Tomatoes
Turnip and other greens

Most other fruits and vegetables contain some vitamin C; fish and milk contain small amounts.

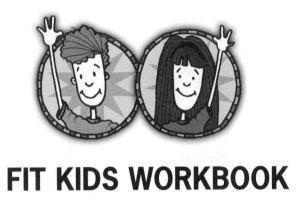

FIT KIDS WORKBOOK

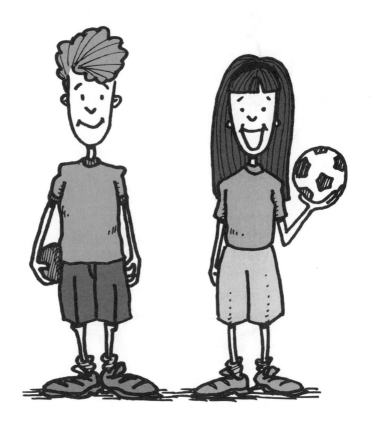

YOU CAN BE A FIT KID, TOO!

Hi! We are the Fit Kids! We take good care of our bodies so that we can play, have fun and do all the cool stuff we like to do. So come along, and you can learn to be a Fit Kid, too!

Parents, the fun activities in this workbook are about the important stuff you are learning in *Raising Fit Kids in a Fat World*. At the bottom of some activities, we list the corresponding chapter from your book so that you can help your kid figure it all out!

We hope you have lots of fun together!

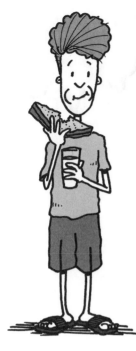

GOD MADE YOU

Do you want to know something really great? God made my body—and yours, too! Crack the code below by using the key to find a letter of the alphabet that matches each symbol. When you are done, you will find out a cool secret about your body!

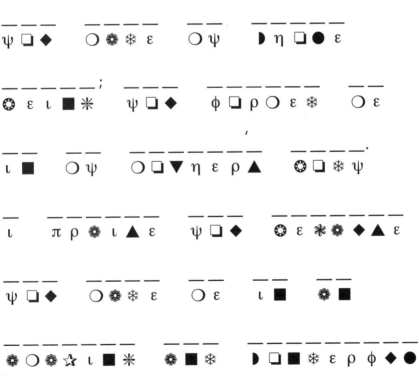

ψ □ ◆   ○ ✿ ❄ ε   ○ ψ   ) η □ ● ε

✿ ε ι ■ ❄ ;   ψ □ ◆   φ □ ρ ○ ε ❄   ○ ε

ι ■   ○ ψ   ○ □ ▼ η ε ρ ▲   ✿ □ ❄ ψ

ι   π ρ ✿ ι ▲ ε   ψ □ ◆   ✿ ε ❄ ✿ ◆ ▲ ε

ψ □ ◆   ○ ✿ ❄ ε   ○ ε   ι ■   ✿ ■

✿ ○ ✿ ☆ ι ■ ❄   ✿ ■ ❄   ) □ ■ ❄ ε ρ φ ◆ ●

) ✿ ψ . (Psalm 139:13-14)

GOD MADE YOU SYMBOL KEY

❀	◎	✳	❄	ε	φ	✳	η	ι
a	b	c	d	e	f	g	h	i

φ	κ	●	○	■	❑	π	θ	ρ
j	k	l	m	n	o	p	q	r

▲	▼	◆	❖	◗	ξ	ψ	☆
s	t	u	v	w	x	y	z

 ANSWER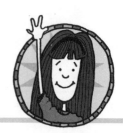

You made my whole being; you formed me in my mother's body. I praise you because you made me in an amazing and wonderful way.

YOU ARE SPECIAL!

In the picture below there is a hidden message! See if you can find all of the letters that spell out:

GOD MADE ME SPECIAL

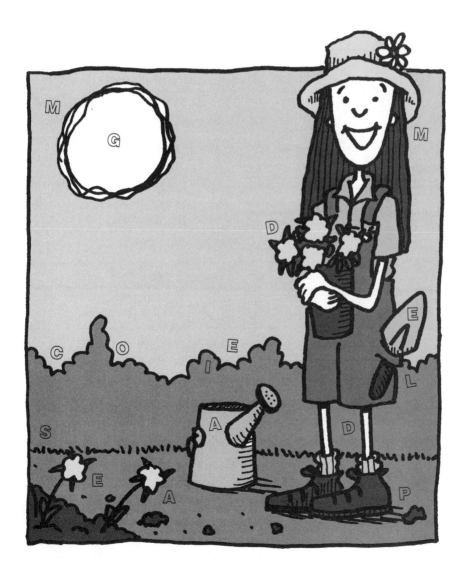

SPECIAL THINGS ABOUT ME:

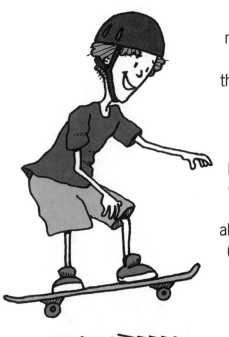

When God designed you, he made you UNIQUE. That means that there are lots of special things about you. Nobody else in the whole world is exactly like you. You are one of a kind. In fact, you are God's master-piece! The way you look is just one little tiny part of the whole you. List some special things about yourself on the lines below (ask your mom or dad for help if you need to!).

_____

_____

_____

_____

_____

_____

_____

_____

_____

EATING THE RIGHT AMOUNT

An important part of becoming a Fit Kid is to make sure that you eat the right amount of food. Did you know that when God made your body, He put special signals inside that tell you when to eat and when to stop? That's why even itty-bitty babies know when they are hungry and full. But sometimes, we don't listen to what our tummies are saying, and then we eat too much food.

LOOK AT EACH BALLOON AND PRETEND IT IS YOUR STOMACH.

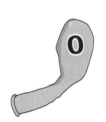

When the balloon is completely EMPTY, like when you first take it out of the package, that is what an empty stomach looks like. We sometimes call this being at a 0. When your stomach gets EMPTY or at a 0, it is time to eat!

When the balloon starts to stretch a little and gets nice and round, it means your stomach is SATIS-FIED. A satisfied stomach, or a stomach at a 5, is about the size of your fist. When your stomach gets to this point, you aren't hungry anymore. If you keep eating past a 5, you will soon feel full or stuffed, and that means you ate too much! When your stomach is SATISFIED or at a 5, it is time to stop eating!

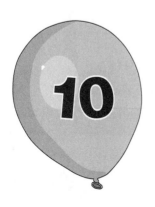

If the balloon gets really stretched out, like it's about to pop, that is what your stomach looks like when you eat too much! We sometimes call that being at a 10. Look out . . . you're going to have a stomach ache soon! If your stomach feels really FULL or you feel like you need to unbutton your jeans, that means you ate too much, and next time you might want to stop eating sooner. (Don't worry—your stomach will never pop!)

WHEN IS THE RIGHT TIME?

Using the Word Bank at the side of the page, fill in the blanks below to describe how you know when it is time to start eating, time to stop eating, or when you might have eaten too much.

I know it is time to eat when:

1. _____
   _____

2. _____
   _____

3. _____
   _____

I know it is time to stop eating when:

1. _____
   _____

2. _____
   _____

3. _____
   _____

I know I ate too much when:

1. _____
   _____

2. _____
   _____

3. _____
   _____

Word BanK

- My stomach feels full, stuffed or about to pop.

- My stomach feels just right.

- My stomach feels completely empty.

- My stomach feels like a nice, round balloon.

- I feel sick to my stomach.

- My stomach doesn't feel hungry anymore.

- My stomach is like an empty balloon.

- My stomach feels hungry even when I'm busy doing something fun.

- I feel like I need to loosen my pants or lie down.

PARENTS:
Read chapters 3 and 4 for more information on hunger and fullness.

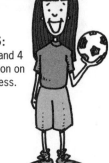

WHAT IS YOUR STOMACH TELLING YOU

DRAW A CIRCLE around the pictures and words below that help you pay attention to what your stomach is telling you about being hungry or satisfied. DRAW AN X over the pictures and words that make it harder to listen to what your stomach is saying.

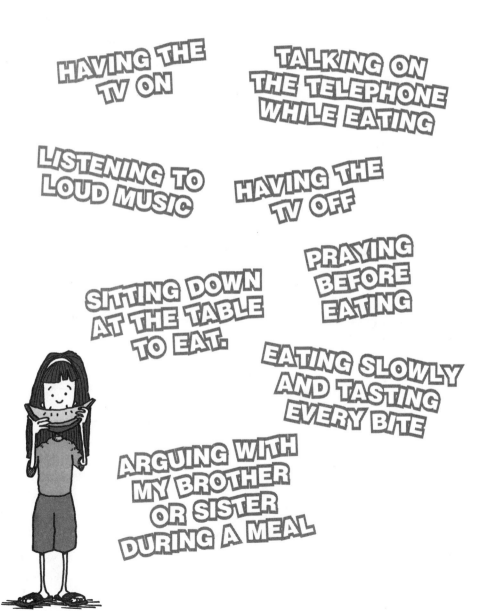

HAVING THE TV ON

TALKING ON THE TELEPHONE WHILE EATING

LISTENING TO LOUD MUSIC

HAVING THE TV OFF

SITTING DOWN AT THE TABLE TO EAT.

PRAYING BEFORE EATING

EATING SLOWLY AND TASTING EVERY BITE

ARGUING WITH MY BROTHER OR SISTER DURING A MEAL

GOD MADE YOU JUST THE RIGHT SIZE

Did you know that when God designed your body, He made it to be just the right size? Our bodies work best when they are the size He designed for us. If you don't eat enough of the right stuff, your body can't grow right and will be too thin. That means you might not have enough energy to do the fun stuff you want to do. If you eat too much food, your body may get too heavy. That makes it hard to run around without getting tired and to get up and down off the floor easily. But eating the RIGHT STUFF in the RIGHT AMOUNTS and BEING ACTIVE EVERY DAY will help your body be just the size God made it to be!

DRAW A CIRCLE around the boxes below that will help your body be just the right size:

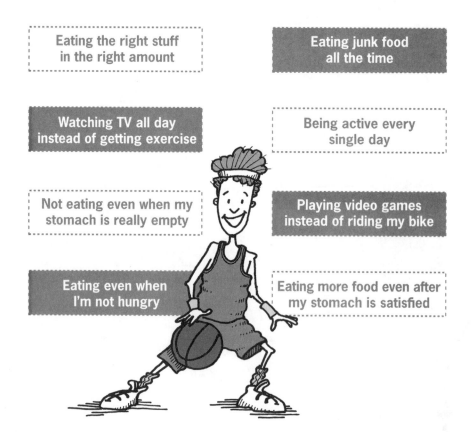

Eating the right stuff in the right amount

Eating junk food all the time

Watching TV all day instead of getting exercise

Being active every single day

Not eating even when my stomach is really empty

Playing video games instead of riding my bike

Eating even when I'm not hungry

Eating more food even after my stomach is satisfied

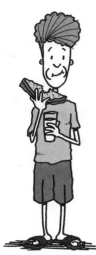

CRACK THE CODE

Crack the code below to find out eight secrets that can help you pay attention to your stomach and eat the right amount of food. Use the key to match each symbol to a letter of the alphabet.

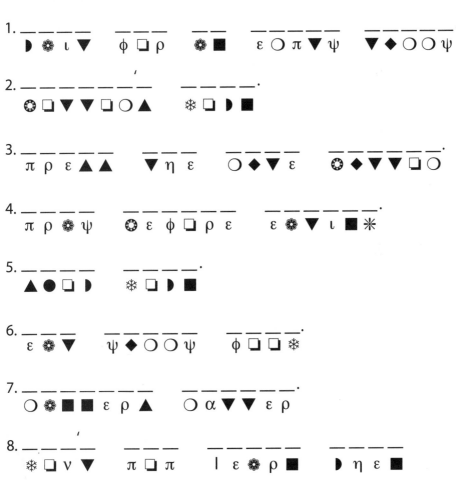

1. ▷ ❀ ι ▼   φ ❑ ρ   ❀ ■   ε ○ π ▼ ψ   ▼ ◆ ○ ○ ψ .

2. ❂ ❑ ▼ ▼ ❑ ○ ▲ ' ❋ ❑ ▷ ■ .

3. π ρ ε ▲ ▲   ▼ η ε   ○ ◆ ▼ ε   ❂ ◆ ▼ ▼ ❑ ○ .

4. π ρ ❀ ψ   ❂ ε φ ❑ ρ ε   ε ❀ ▼ ι ■ ❋ .

5. ▲ ● ❑ ▷   ❋ ❑ ▷ ■ .

6. ε ❀ ▼   ψ ◆ ○ ○ ψ   φ ❑ ❑ ❋ .

7. ○ ❀ ■ ■ ε ρ ▲   ○ α ▼ ▼ ε ρ .

8. ❋ ❑ ν ▼   π ❑ π   ι ε ❀ ρ ■   ▷ η ε ■

   ▼ ❑   ▲ ▼ ❑ π .

CRACK THE CODE SYMBOL KEY

❀	❂	✳	❄	ε	φ	✳	η	ι
a	b	c	d	e	f	g	h	i

φ	κ	●	○	■	❑	π	θ	ρ
j	k	l	m	n	o	p	q	r

▲	▼	◆	❖	◗	ξ	ψ	☆
s	t	u	v	w	x	y	z

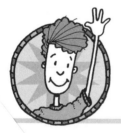 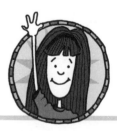

ANSWERS

1. Wait for an empty tummy.
2. Bottom's down.
3. Press the mute button.
4. Pray before eating.
5. Slow down.
6. Eat yummy food.
7. Manners Matter
8. Don't pop learn when to stop.

EATING THE RIGHT STUFF

Once you have gotten the hang of eating the **right amount**, your next important job is to learn how to eat the **right stuff**. Food is really important, because it provides important things called NUTRIENTS to help your body work better. Did you know that by eating the right stuff, you can make your bones stronger and get well quicker when you are sick? VITAMINS and MINERALS are some of the nutrients in food, and they have important jobs inside your body. Unscramble the words below to discover which foods contain these important vitamins.

VITAMIN A

_ _ _ _
segg

_ _ _ _
eatm

_ _ _ _ _ _
eeesch

_ _ _ _
evlir

VITAMIN K

_ _ _ _ _ _ _
bbageca

_ _ _ _ _ _ _ _ _ _
reluacifolw

_ _ _ _ _ _ _
niacshp

_ _ _ _ _ _ _ _
ysnasobe

VITAMIN D

_ _ _ _ _ _
tebutr

_ _ _ _
hfis

_ _ _ _ _ _
syteor

_ _ _ _ _ _
aelecr

VITAMIN E

_ _ _ _ _ _ _ _
htaew mgre

_ _ _ _ _
leoiv

_ _ _ _ _ _ _
hcinspa

_ _ _ _ _ _ _ _ _
psarasuga

PARENTS:
To find out more information about vitamins and minerals, the important roles they play in our bodies and their main food sources, read chapter 5 and appendix C.

Vitamin A: eggs, meat, cheese, liver. **Vitamin D:** butter, fish, oyster, cereal. **Vitamin E:** wheat germ, olive, spinach, asparagus. **Vitamin K:** cabbage, cauliflower, spinach, soybeans.

WHAT DO VITAMINS DO?

Can you guess what vitamins and minerals do?
To find out, use the key to fill in each vitamin
that matches a symbol in the blanks below.

Vitamin A=✹   Vitamin B2=✪   Vitamin B3=✳

Vitamin B6=✳   Vitamin C=✳   Vitamin D=✳

Vitamin B12=✳   Vitamin K=✳   Folic Acid=✲

These vitamins keep my eyes healthy.

1. _____   2. _____
         ✹   ✪

These vitamins give me healthy skin.

1. _____   2. _____   3. _____
         ✹   ✪   ✳

4. _____
         ✳

This vitamin helps my body to heal and resist infection.

1. _____
         ✳

These vitamins help my body to produce blood and help blood to clot.

1. _____   2. _____   3. _____
         ✳   ✳   ✲

4. _____   5. _____
         ✳   ✲

These vitamins help me grow.

1. _____   2. _____   3. _____
         ✹   ✳   ✳

WHOLE-BODY PLEASERS

When food tastes good but doesn't really satisfy you or do anything to help your body work better, that food is called a TASTE BUD-TEASER. When food tastes good, makes your stomach feel satisfied AND has nutrients in it that help your body work better, that food is called a WHOLE-BODY PLEASER. Play the matching game below to help learn the difference!

Sugary treats that
taste great but don't really
fill up my stomach

**TASTE-BUD
TEASER**

My favorite fruit that
tastes yummy

**WHOLE-BODY
PLEASER**

Food that tastes great,
satisfies my stomach and
is good for my body

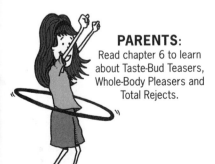

PARENTS:
Read chapter 6 to learn
about Taste-Bud Teasers,
Whole-Body Pleasers and
Total Rejects.

Food that comes in
a cool package,
but my dad calls it
"junk food"

A meal that Mom
cooks at home that
she says is good
for me

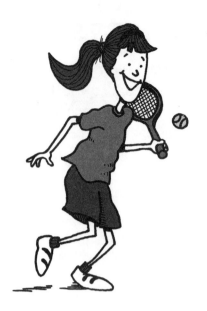

Now that you know the difference between Taste-Bud Teasers and Whole-Body Pleasers, list some of each in the spaces below. Ask your mom or dad to help you decide.

TASTE-BUD TEASER

WHOLE-BODY PLEASER

GET MOVING!

Another really important part of being a FIT KID is being ACTIVE. Circle the words in the puzzle below to discover some ways to HAVE FUN and BE FIT all at the same time!

L	M	R	K	B	E	B	O	W	L	I	N	G
L	E	O	F	A	M	I	L	Y	W	A	L	K
A	I	L	R	S	W	C	E	C	R	I	T	A
T	O	L	I	E	I	Y	L	O	T	I	S	R
E	N	E	G	B	H	C	G	J	I	L	N	A
N	W	R	K	A	E	L	S	U	B	O	A	T
N	C	S	B	L	C	I	L	M	I	O	E	E
I	B	K	M	L	I	N	S	P	H	T	T	E
S	C	A	V	E	N	G	E	R	H	U	N	T
N	P	T	S	T	V	B	L	O	H	A	C	O
S	W	I	M	M	I	N	G	P	L	I	L	M
L	U	N	F	R	I	S	B	E	E	B	A	L
P	O	G	O	S	T	I	C	K	N	R	E	F

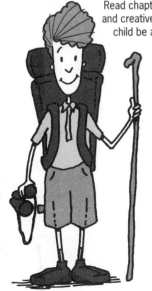

PARENTS:
Read chapter 7 for lots of fun and creative ways to help your child be active every day.

WORD LIST
Baseball
Frisbee
Bowling
Karate
Bicycling
Ballet
Family Walk
Pogo Stick
Scavenger Hunt
Roller Skating
Jump Rope
Tennis
Swimming

HEART HUNGER AND STOMACH HUNGER

Have you ever noticed that sometimes you eat even though you aren't hungry? Sometimes the reason we do that is because our HEART is hungry. Read below (or have your mom or dad read aloud) to find out the difference between a hungry STOMACH and a hungry HEART.

Heart Hunger

HEART HUNGER means that something is bothering you on the inside. It might mean that you are mad, sad, bored, scared or frustrated. Or you might feel like no one is paying attention to you. Sometimes it might even mean that something good happened and you want to celebrate and reward yourself. When your heart is hungry, food doesn't help. FOOD is for STOMACH hunger only.

Stomach Hunger

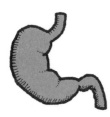

STOMACH HUNGER is what you feel when your stomach is completely empty or at a 0. It doesn't have anything to do with whether you are happy or sad. Most people's stomachs feel hungry right above the belly button and maybe just a little to the left side. It might feel empty or hollow, and might even make a growling noise! When your stomach is really hungry, it is time to eat!

PARENTS:
Read chapter 9 to learn more about heart hunger and your child's deepest longings.

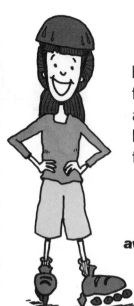

Read the sentences below about how you might feel at different times. Then draw a SQUARE around each sentence that describes HEART HUNGER. Draw a CIRCLE around each sentence that describes STOMACH HUNGER.

I made a bad grade on my math test and it made me feel really sad and mad.

I woke up and got dressed, and then I heard my stomach growling!

My team won the championship and I felt like having a big celebration!

Mom and Dad were mad at each other and arguing, and that made me feel scared and lonely.

When I got home from school, I felt like my stomach was completely empty.

My best friend asked someone else to play with her today and didn't invite me. That hurt my feelings.

It rained all day and I didn't have anything to do.

After playing outside, a place inside my stomach right above my belly button felt hungry.

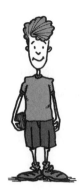
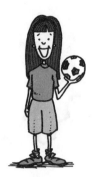

FIT KID PATHWAY

On the next page is the FIT KID PATHWAY for you to follow over the next few days! Start today at the beginning of the pathway. When you make a choice that helps you become a FIT KID, you get to move forward! The FIT KID CHOICES are listed below along with how many spaces you can move ahead for each choice. To mark your spot, draw a star or a smiley face, or maybe your mom or dad will help you find some cool stickers. When you reach the finish line, ask your mom or dad for a prize!

MOVE 1 SPACE FORWARD WHEN YOU:
- Drink water or milk at one meal
- Turn off all noisy things (like the TV) when eating today
- Take the stairs instead of the elevator
- Wait for an empty stomach before eating
- Stop eating at 5, BEFORE getting full
- Try a new fruit
- Try a new vegetable
- Do 20 jumping jacks
- Play outside for 30 minutes
- Ride your bike after dinner
- Mom or Dad's suggestions: _____ _____

MOVE 3 SPACES FORWARD WHEN YOU:
- Play outside for an hour
- Substitute a Whole-Body Pleaser for a Taste-Bud Teaser
- Drink water or milk at every meal
- Jump rope for 30 minutes
- Watch LESS than 1 hour of TV today
- Go all day without drinking a cola or sugary drink
- Eat meals at the dinner table for a whole week
- Are active indoors for an hour
- Do something OTHER than eating to help your hungry heart feel better
- Eat fruit and vegetables at every meal for a week
- Mom or Dad's suggestions: _____ _____

FIT KID PATHWAY

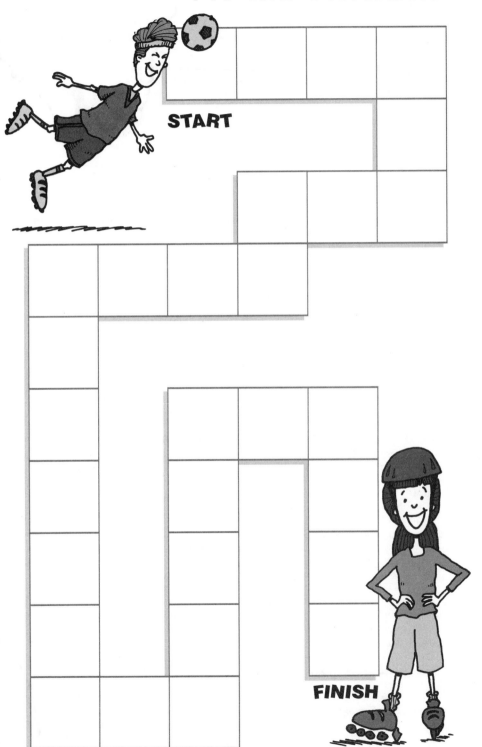

START

FINISH

ENDNOTES

Chapter 1: Have Hope!
1. Walt Larimore, M.D., "Generation XL," *Parents* (March 2007), pp. 8-9.
2. Stephen Daniels, "The Consequences of Childhood Overweight and Obesity," *The Future of Children: Childhood Obesity*, vol. 16, no. 1 (2006), pp. 47-67. Visit www.futureofchildren.org.
3. S. A. Richardson, N. Goodman, A. H. Hastorf, et al, "Cultural Uniformity in Reaction to Physical Disabilities," *American Sociological Review*, vol. 26 (1961), pp. 241-247.

Chapter 2: Getting Oriented
1. N. F. Krebs and M. S. Jacobson, "Prevention of Pediatric Overweight and Obesity," *Pediatrics*, vol. 112, no. 2 (2003), pp. 424-430.
2. M. Golan, A. Weizman, A. Apter, et al, "Parents as the Exclusive Agents of Change in the Treatment of Childhood Obesity," *American Journal of Clinical Nutrition*, vol. 67 (1998), pp. 1130-1135.
3. "BMI—Body Mass Index: About BMI for Children and Teens," Centers for Disease Control and Prevention, Department of Health and Human Services. http://www.cdc.gov/nccd php/dnpa/bmi/childrens_BMI/about_childrens_BMI.htm (accessed June 2007).
4. Judy Halliday, *Thin Within* (Nashville: W Publishing Group, 2002), p. 59.
5. A. A. Hedley, C. L. Ogden, C. L. Johnson, et al, "Overweight and Obesity Among US Children, Adolescents, and Adults 1999-2002," *JAMA*, vol. 291 (2004), pp. 2847-2850.
6. Lara Trifiletti, Wendy Shields, et al, "Tipping the Scales: Obese Children and Child Safety Seats," *Pediatrics*, vol. 117, no. 4 (2006), pp. 1197-1202.
7. William H. Dietz, "Health Consequences of Obesity in Youth: Childhood Predictors of Adult Disease," *Pediatrics*, vol. 101 (1998), pp. 518-525.
8. S. Mustillo, C. Worthman, A. Erkanli, et al, "Obesity and Psychiatric Disorder: Developmental Trajectories," *Pediatrics*, vol. 111, no. 4 (2003), pp. 851-859.

Chapter 3: Hunger and Fullness
1. L. Young and M. Nestle, "The Contribution of Expanding Portion Sizes to the US Obesity Epidemic, *American Journal of Public Health,* vol. 92, no. 2 (2002), pp. 246-249.
2. N. Diliberti, P. Bordi, M. Conklin, et al, "Increased Portion Size Leads to Increased Energy Intake in a Restaurant Meal," *Obesity Research*, vol. 12, no. 3 (2004), pp. 562-568.

Chapter 4: Ages and Stages
1. L. M. Gartner, R. A. Lawrence and A. J. Naylor, "Breastfeeding and the Use of Human Milk," *Pediatrics*, vol. 115, no. 2 (2005), pp. 496-506.
2. Ibid.
3. Catarina Canivet, Irene Jakobsson and Barbro Hagander, "Colicky Infants According to Maternal Reports in Telephone Interviews and Diaries: A Large Scandinavian Study," *Developmental and Behavioral Pediatrics*, vol. 23, no. 1 (2002), pp. 1-8.
4. A. Fiocchi, A. Assa'ad and S. Bahna, "Food Allergy and the Introduction of Solid Foods to Infants: A Consensus Document. Adverse Reactions to Foods Committee, American College of Allergy, Asthma and Immunology," *Annals of Allergy, Asthma and Clinical Immunology*, vol. 97, no. 1 (2006), pp. 10-20.
5. Erma Bombeck, *Forever Erma* (New York: Fawcett Books, 1996), p. 20.
6. Charles Swindoll, *Parenting: From Surviving to Thriving* (Nashville: W Publishing Group, 2006), p. xv, emphasis added.

Chapter 5: Get Smart About Food Facts
1. *Merriam-Webster's Medical Dictionary*, s.v., "healthy." http://dictionary.reference.com/browse/healthy (accessed January 2007).
2. "Building Blocks for Fun and Healthy Meals—A Menu Planner for the Child and Adult Care Food Program," United States Department of Agriculture Food and Nutrition Service, Spring 2000. http://www.fns.usda.gov/tn/Resources/buildingblocks.html (accessed June 2007).

3. Mitch Lazar, M.D., Ph.D., "Insulin Resistance." Paper presented at Stanford University School of Medicine, March 1, 2007.
4. "My Pyramid Plan," United States Department of Agriculture. http://www.mypyramid.gov/index.html (accessed June 2007).

Chapter 6: Smarts in Action

1. Betterfoodchoices.com, "Most TV Food Ads Send the Wrong Message to Kids." http://www.betterfoodchoices.com/news_detail.php?NewsArticleID=9 (accessed June 2007).
2. Grace Wyshak, "Teenaged Girls, Carbonated Beverage Consumption, and Bone Fractures," *Archives of Pediatrics and Adolescent Medicine*, vol. 154, no. 6 (2000), pp. 610-613.
3. Katherine L. Tucker, Kyoko Morita, Ning Qiao, et al, "Colas, But Not Other Carbonated Beverages, Are Associated with Low Bone Mineral Density in Older Women: The Framingham Osteoporosis Study," *American Journal of Clinical Nutrition*, vol. 84 (2006), pp. 936-942.

Chapter 7: Get a Move On

1. B. Marcus, D. Williams, P. Dubbert, et al, "Physical Activity Intervention Studies: What We Know and What We Need to Know: A Scientific Statement from the American Heart Association Council on Nutrition, Physical Activity, and Metabolism (Subcommittee on Physical Activity); Council on Cardiovascular Disease in the Young; and the Interdisciplinary Working Group on Quality of Care and Outcomes Research," *Circulation*, vol. 114 (2006), pp. 2739-2752.
2. K. J. Calfas and W. C. Taylor, "Effects of Physical Activity on Psychological Variables in Adolescents," *Pediatric Exercise Science*, vol. 6 (1994), pp. 406-423.
3. American Academy of Pediatrics Policy Statement, Council on Sports Medicine and Fitness and Council on School Health, "Active Healthy Living: Prevention of Childhood Obesity Through Increased Physical Activity," *Pediatrics*, vol. 117 (May 2006), pp. 1834-1842.
4. R. E. Andersen, C. J. Crespo, S. J. Bartlett, et al, "Relationship of Physical Activity and Television Watching with Body Weight and Level of Fatness Among Children: Results from the Third National Health and Nutrition Examination Survey," *JAMA*, vol. 279 (1998), pp. 938 -942.
5. Centers for Disease Control and Prevention, "Physical Activity Levels Among Children Aged 9-13 years: United States, 2002," *MMWR, Morbidity and Mortality Weekly Report*, vol. 52 (2003), pp. 785 -788.

Chapter 9: Hungry Hearts

1. Charles Swindoll, *Parenting: From Surviving to Thriving* (Nashville, TN: W Publishing Group, 2006), p. 67.

Chapter 10: Obstacle Course

1. Max Lucado, *In the Eye of the Storm* (Nashville, TN: Word Publishing, 1991), p. 11.
2. *WordNet 2.0, Farlex clipart collection.* s.v., "saboteur," http://www.thefreedictionary.com/saboteur (accessed June 2007).
3. W. H. Dietz, Jr., and S. L. Dortmaker, "Do We Fatten Our Children at the Television Set?" *Pediatrics*, vol. 75 (1985), pp. 807-812.
4. "Prayer Attributed to Civil War Soldier," at HolisticOnline.com. http://1stholistic.com/Spl_prayers/prayer_civilwar.htm (accessed June 2007).

Chapter 12: A Time to Soar

1. Erma Bombeck, *Forever Erma* (Kansas City: Andrews and McCeel, Kansas City, 1996), p. xiii.
2. *Chariots of Fire*, directed by Hugh Hudson. Edinburgh, Scotland: Enigma Productions, 1981.

Appendix

1. Department of Health and Human Services, "Body mass index-for-age percentiles: Girls, 2 to 20 years 5th, 10th, 25th, 50th, 75th, 85th, 90th, 95th percentiles," Centers for Disease Control and Prevention. http://www.cdc.gov/nchs/data/nhanes/growthcharts/set2/chart%2016.pdf (accessed June 2007). Shading added.
2. *MedLine Plus*, s.v., "vitamins." http://www.nlm.nih.gov/medlineplus/ency/article/002399.htm (accessed June 2007).

ACKNOWLEDGMENTS

There are so many who helped contribute to this project that it is impossible to acknowledge all of our friends, helpers, prayer warriors and counselors that God placed in our path.

Heidi Byslma receives our heartfelt gratitude. Her creative writing, wisdom and life experiences greatly enriched this book. Her willingness to jump in at the last minute and pour her heart into this project turned a monumental task into a joyful experience. Words are inadequate to express our appreciation for your generous contribution, beloved friend.

Mark Sweeney, our agent, and his lovely wife, Janet, deserve our sincere thanks for being faithful servants of God and for their patience, guidance and friendship. We are also thankful to all those at Regal for their amazing gifts, hard work and commitment to Christ.

Judy thankfully acknowledges:
The many Thin Within participants whose testimonies are woven throughout the pages of this book, including our faithful friends Susan Ford, Pam Sneed, Lisa Cauto and Jan Tabrizi, who supported us with their valuable input and steadfast prayers; Allie Smith, my youthful friend who is wise beyond her years and whose feedback was received with sincere gratitude; Sheila Kogan, my precious sister in the Lord, who freely gave of her wisdom and insight in the early stages of the manuscript.

Jennifer Jansons, whose cheerful spirit, keen eye and computer skills made it possible for us to meet a demanding deadline; my dear sister Colette, whose consistent prayers and faith in God's equipping power carried us to the finish line; and our ministry partners and dear friends Joe and Pam Donaldson, whose management of the Thin Within ministry made it possible for us to write this book.

High praises to my beloved husband, Arthur, for his invaluable editing skills, patience and partnership throughout the entire project. Couldn't have done it without you, my love!

Most of all, I give my highest praise to our Lord Jesus Christ. It is only through much prayer and total dependency on the Spirit that this book was written. To Him we give all of the honor and glory!

Joani gratefully acknowledges:
Mike, my husband and best friend, for your willingness to do whatever was needed; for being a single dad during the months before the deadline; for providing extra love and attention to the girls when I didn't have much left; for your amazing research skills; for making the workbook happen; and for your unfailing love, prayers and support. I love you and thank God every day for you.

My girls, Jessica and Gracie, for your love and prayers, for giving me peace and quiet when needed, for allowing me to use your stories, and for all the hugs and kisses that kept me going. Being with you gives me a glimpse of the face of God, and I love you bunches.

My family and friends who willingly dropped whatever they were doing to pray, offer heartfelt advice, read the manuscript or simply put up with me: Charles Barnes (Dad), Brenda and Tom Williams, Steve and Debbie Barnes, Tim Filston, Ardith Kilgore, Dr. Bill Dudley (beloved pastor), Maribeth Powers, Tony and Jenny Nash, Sandy and Garth Whitcombe, Douglas Word, Chuck Barnes, Sleepy and Jane Jack, Kathy Jack, Dr. Susan Hayes (my very first coauthor), Dr. Chuck Tigar and Dr. Yolanda Spraggins.

My ladies' small group at Signal Mountain Presbyterian Church (the Youth Group): Mary Adams, Donna Curry, Debbie Garvich, Jane Harris, Joy Ludwig, Ruth Maxwell, Joan McCandless, Anne McElhinny, Phyllis Roberts, Mary Lynn Shelton, Deane Sprague, Milissa Westbrook and Sharon Woods. Thanks so much for your constant prayers, support and friendship.

My patients and their parents, who have taught me so much, for your trust and for sharing your lives with me.

Most of all, thank You, Jesus, my Lord and my God. You have blessed me beyond measure. Please, Lord, use this book to Your glory.

NOTE FROM THE AUTHORS

We love to hear from our readers! You can contact us at:

Judy Halliday/Thin Within
P.O Box 1438
Los Altos, CA 94023
Toll Free number: (877) 729-8932
www.thinwithin.org

Dr. Joani Jack
P.O. Box 724
Signal Mountain, TN 37377
joanijackmd@yahoo.com

Do you wish there was an approach for Raising *Fit Adults* in a Fat World?

There is!!

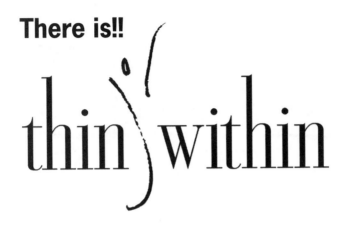

Check out *Thin Within*,
the original hunger-fullness guide to making wise food choices as you melt down to your natural size. A ministry started by Judy Halliday in 1975.

○ Grace oriented approach
○ Not another diet
○ Dynamic Bible study
○ Great for groups or individuals

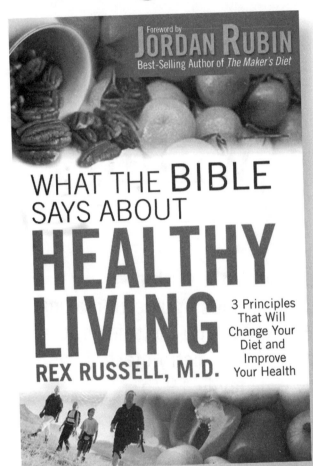
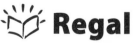